new practitioners in the future health service

explori

nary and

interm

edited

ippr 2002

1 86030 206 8

ippr
30-32 Southampton Street
London
WC2E 7RA
tel +44 (0)20 7470 6100
fax +44 (0)20 7470 6111
email info@ippr.org.uk
www.ippr.org.uk

charity number: 800065

ippr is the leading independent think tank on the centre left. Through our well-researched and clearly argued policy analysis, our publications, and our strong networks in government, academia and the corporate and voluntary sectors, we play a vital role in maintaining the momentum of progressive thought.

Contents

Contents

Acknowledgements

With grateful thanks to Tania Meyer (LSE) and Sarah Deacon (IPPR) for their help in editing and disseminating the papers. Thanks also to the sponsors of the Future Health Worker project: Boots The Chemists, Pfizer, PRIME and Lloydspharmacy.

About the Contributors

Stephen Fishwick is National Campaigns Manager at Diabetes UK, Europe's largest patient organisation. In this role, he is responsible for promoting the patient voice in the development and implementation of the forthcoming diabetes National Service Framework. Previously he worked as a political consultant in the energy sector, having begun his career, abroad, in education. His published articles and pamphlets range from *Advocacy and Health Economics* (2001) to *Who's New? Young People in Today's Labour Party* (1996).

Liz Kendall is an Associate Director at IPPR and responsible for running the Institute's programme of research on health and social care. She was previously the Fellow of the Public Health Programme at the King's Fund and, from 1996-1998, a Special Adviser to the Rt Hon Harriet Harman, MP, Secretary of State for Social Security and Minister for Women. Liz's most recent publications include *From Welfare to Wellbeing: the future of social care* (2002) and *The Future Patient* (2001).

Melinda Letts has worked for 20 years in non-profit organisations, including eleven years in the health sector. She is Chairwoman of the Long Term Medical Conditions Alliance, an alliance of 115 voluntary health organisations which promotes the shared needs and concerns of people living with long-term illness. She is also Deputy Chair of Trustees of the General Practice Airways Group, a Commissioner with the Commission for Health Improvement, and a member of the NHS Modernisation Board.

Rachel Lissauer is a Research Fellow in Health Policy at the IPPR. She is the lead researcher for the Future Health Worker project and was previously a member of the secretariat for IPPR's Commission on Public Private Partnerships where she carried out the Commission's work on PPPs in health and education. Her previous publications include *Building Better Partnerships* (2001); *PPPs in Primary Care* (2000) and *A Learning Process: public private partnerships in education* (2000).

Andrew Murdock is Pharmacy Director and Superintendent Pharmacist for Lloydspharmacy. He sits on the National Pharmaceutical Association Board, is a member of the Pharmaceutical Services Negotiating Committee and the Company Chemists' Association, and is a Director of the Pharmacy Healthcare Scheme, as well as being an external advisor to Bradford University's School of Pharmacy. He writes here in a personal capacity.

Cecilia Pyper is a National Primary Care Career Scientist in the Health Services Research Unit, Department of Public Health, Universituy of Oxford, where she also tutors in primary care. She is a part-time GO at Bury Knowle Health Centre, Oxford. Her specialist interests include reproductive health, community participation and more recently, user access to electronic health reconrds. She has been a consultant to the US Agency for Interational Development and the International Planned Parenthood Federation. Currently she is is investigating NHS professional and patient access to online electronic health records for the Deprtment of Health and NHS Information Authority.

Ruth Tennant was formerly a programme manager on the Public Health Programme at the King's Fund where she has worked on a range of issues including the future of public health, patient and public involvement and health and London governance. Ruth was previously research and policy advisor to the Controller of the Audit Commission and has also worked in the European Parliament and as a non executive director of Southwark primary care trust. She is now a public health specialist on the West Midlands training scheme.

Barbara Vaughan is an independent consultant with experience of working in practice, education, research and development. She led the King's Fund Intermediate Care Programme and has been responsible for supporting local developments, national debate and a series of publications in this area. Barbara is a non-executive director for her local PCT with a lead for implementation of the NSF for Older People.

David Woodhead is Fellow in Health Policy at the King's Fund. He has worked across the health economy (in the NHS, local government and the voluntary sector) and in a number of academic institutions. His current work addresses inequalities through policy analysis, research and partnership development.

Jeremy Wyatt is Director of the Knowledge Management Centre, School of Public Policy, UCL and visiting professor in medical informatics, Academic Medical Centre, University of Amsterdam. After training and practising as a physician he became involved in the evidence-based medicine movement, helping set up the Cochrane Collaboration in 1992 and designing software to help doctors carry out better quality trials. He has written three Lancet series on clinical knowledge, clinical data systems, and information design and a 10-article series on Knowledge for the Clinician.

1. INTRODUCTION

Rachel Lissauer and Liz Kendall

The Future Health Worker project aims to explore the implications for health service staff of providing care that is 'patient-centred'. It builds on the understanding of patients' likely needs and expectations over the next five to fifteen years, that was developed within an earlier ippr study, *The Future Patient* (Kendall 2001). This argued that, whilst the majority of patients value the NHS and want to see a public health service continue, too many are dissatisfied with the treatment they receive. Patients struggle to gain quick and convenient access to healthcare, to find services which meet their needs in the round and to get the information and relationships with practitioners they need to participate as active and equal partners in their own care.

The Future Health Worker project has sought to address how health practioners' roles will need to change in order to address these shortcomings. This pamphlet aims to provide a 'snapshot' of some of the new roles and types of practitioners that should be considered as part of the process of making care patient-centred. Each paper sets out the role of a particular type or types of practitioner: an intermediate care practitioner; a 'telecarer', a knowledge broker, a 'lay' practitioner, a consultant pharmacist and a public health leader. The authors outline the essential features of each role, explore how the 'new' practitioner would aid the provision of more patient-focused care and then considers the policy changes needed in order to aid their development.

New practitioners and the provision of patient-centred care

Timely and convenient access

A critical feature of patent centred health services is that they provide timely and convenient access to care. There is a plethora of evidence that the public's top concern with the NHS is waiting for treatment. For example, whilst surveys indicate a positive response from patients to primary care services overall, difficulties with getting an appointment with a GP are a key source of dissatisfaction (Audit Commission, 2002; Exley and Jarvis, 2001). As more people work longer hours, demand for quicker and more convenient access to treatment will grow. An increasinly 24/7 culture means patients now expect more flexible access to healthcare, including access to services outside traditional working hours (Cabinet Office, 2000). The NHS is beginning to respond to these demands. NHS Direct, the nurse-led telephone helpline is expected to manage 30 million calls a year by 2008; nurse-led triage is being used in accident and emergency departments to reduce waiting times; and nurse practitioners are improving access to primary care.

So the means of accessing health services are already changing. The notion that GPs will not necessarily be 'the first port of call' for the health service, whilst by no means universally supported, is now widely acknowledged. Yet the changes in roles of primary care practitioners should not be restricted to considerations of where nurses are able to 'substitute' for doctors. The goal of improving access should be seen as part of a broader aim of ensuring that patients' needs for assessment, diagnosis, treatment and reassurance are met and managed appropriately. The contribution that the wider health service workforce can play, as well the role of patients themselves, must now be better recognised and developed.

Policy-makers and professionals have been discussing the development of community pharmacy services since the Nuffield Report of 1986. Recent policy changes include changes in pharmacists contractual arrangements allowing them to be rewarded for overall service rather than being paid predominantly for the dispensing of individual prescriptions (Department of Health, 2000). Pharmacists' roles in the management of minor injuries, repeat dispensing and health promotion are now being explored throughout the UK (Whittington *et al*, 2001).

However, Andrew Murdock suggests that lack of capacity within the pharmacy workforce is acting as a significant inhibitor to the further extension of pharmacists' roles. He makes the controversial suggestion of 'cleaving' the current role of the pharamcists, both as a possible solution to current capacity constraints and as a means of preparing them for taking on future responsibility, for deciding the appropriate therapy for patients, on the basis of the GP's diagnosis. Murdock suggests the developments of a consultant pharmacist, who would be responsible for medicines management and monitoring and screening patients, and a pharmacy technician (supported by accredited checking technicians) who would be responsible for carrying out routine dispensing. He highlights the calculation that 2.75 million hours of doctors' time could be saved if pharmacists were to control the process of dispensing by installments prescriptions written by a GP for long-term medical conditions. In future, instead of patients having to collect repeat prescriptions from the GP and take them to the pharmacy, they could be contacted directly by pharmacists when they need their medicine or even visited by pharmacists at home. Pharmacists could also monitor patients' health status, check for adverse drug reactions, and screen for previously undiagnosed conditions.

Developing the role of community pharmacists is one way of broadening access to health services and ensuring health needs are more appropriately and effectively met. However, in future patients will not only seek more convenient ways of meeting professionals face-to-face. As information and communication technologies improve, people will seek to communicate with health professionals and the health service via the telephone and the Internet. This may be particularly true of those patients suffering from chronic conditions, whose numbers are set to increase. These patients require ongoing, but usually brief contact with health professionals, rather than infrequent, formal visits to a hospital outpatient department. However, e-mail consultation is still currently rare. Although some specialists use telemedicine to offer consultations in areas such as dermatology and psychiatry, these practitioners receive little training.

Jeremy Wyatt sets out a bold vision for a future telecarer who would expand the ways in which care is provided. The telecarer is 'a health professional who delivers responsive, high quality services and support to remote patients or clients using the most appropriate and accepted communications media, colleagues and information sources'. Wyatt argues that whilst telecaring may be one aspect of a specialists' wider work, interspersed with their direct clinical practice, it will be a distinctive role for which telecarers will need to be appropriately trained, regulated and remunerated. He outlines a hypothetical job description and person specification of a 'telecarer' and explores the possible barriers to the development of this role.

Meeting health needs in the round

Patient centred care acknolwdges pateints needs in the round and, ideally, treats the causes, not just the symptoms, of their problem. One immediate implication for policy makers and professionals is to identify how practitioners can become better equipped to tackle the determinants of ill health.

Ruth Tennant and David Woodhead suggest that new Public Health Leaders could play an important role in this process. Their paper builds on the recognition that, in future, bio-medicine will no longer dominate the practice of public health. The contribution that a far wider range of different practitioners and agencies can play in health promotion and to the reduction of health inequalities will need to be acknowledged and developed. Bringing together practitioners with a range of backgrounds (such as community development, environmental health, housing and health visiting) and ensuring these practitioners work together will require strong and committed public health leaders.

Tennant and Woodhead suggest that these new public health leaders, whose background may not be medical, will be responsible for assessing and meeting the health needs of their local community. The information they collate on health needs will highlight issues such as environment, housing, traffic management and leisure services where 'upstream' intervention might help to reduce morbidity and mortality. Public health leaders will help set up local health improvement targets, shared across all local agencies, mapping out the range of practitioners who contribute to health improvement. They will act as catalysts, supporting other leaders and health champions, for example in local government to improve the health of local people. Woodhead and Tenant highlight the difficulty that Primary Care Trusts (PCTs) are currently experiencing in recruiting to senior-level public health posts and point to solutions such as joint health improvement posts between PCTs and local councils and skill-sharing between neighbouring PCTs, facilitated by public health networks. These measures, they suggest, will need to be supported and championed by strong national leadership and more effective cross-departmental working and sharing of health improvement objectives.

Providing care that meets patients' needs in the round also means ensuring that care is integrated across different sectors and between different tiers of the health service. Too many patients suffer because agencies fail to work together effectively. Increasing medical specialisation can also work against providing seamless and inegated care, since highly specialised professionals can end up taking a reductionist approach by only treating one element of a patient's condition. These failings are particularly pronounced in the care of the elderly, as Barbara Vaughan vividly illustrates. She argues that current methods of classifying and diagnosing older patients, fail to provide an accurate reflection of their needs. One consequence is that the numbers of patients who would benefit from intermediate care is not established. Vaughan argues that the creation of a new intermediate care practitioner, who would draw together elements of current professions such as nursing, occupational therapy and home support, would help better meet the needs of older people who do not need to be in hospital but would benefit from other types of care such as rehabilitation or recuperation.

Informed and empowered patients

A genuinely patient-centred service must facilitate greater involvement of patients in their own healthcare. The dominant stereotype is still of the health professional who talks about rather than with the patient and to whom patients are mainly embodiments of their condition rather than as partners in the provision of their care. The NHS Plan aspires to a future in which 'the NHS becomes a resource that people routinely use every day to help them look after themselves'. The vision is that the NHS should become a service responsible for helping people to maintain their own healthcare, employing practitioners who are skilled at supporting people in the management of aspects of their care.

Stephen Fishwick and Melinda Letts argue that, whilst the role and notion of 'Expert Patients' has been acknowledged by the Government, this has not been accompanied by the kind of comprehensive policy approach needed to expand patients' roles significantly. They outline the role of a hypothetical 'lay practitioner' - a person with a chronic illness who takes responsibility for managing thier condition - and explore how professionals', patients' and managers' roles would need to change to make the 'lay practitioner' a reality.

Cecilia Pyper's paper focuses on a related issue, that of information provision. Underpinning her paper is the principle that citizens must be encouraged to practice health-improving behaviour and self-care and that the production, analysis and dissemination of information is a vital part of this process. Pyper suggests that in future, an information deficit will be replaced by information overload. The challenge for the NHS will lie in ensuring that information is relevant; that patients have equal access to quality information and that information enables patients/citizens to participate safely and actively in self-care. This will require different types of 'Knowledge Brokers' to emerge. Pyper highlights three distinct roles: a 'peer knowledge broker' who helps those of a similar age, condition or background to access relevant information; an 'IT knowledge broker' who helps patients to use IT to find the information they require and an 'expert knowledge broker': a professional who uses their skills and knowledge to produce and develop tailored information. Pyper gives examples, both national and international, of how these roles have emerged and the factors that have contributed towards their success.

Implications for public policy

Workforce planning has traditionally been based on an assumption that tomorrow's health service workforce will comprise the same professional groups, working within the same institutions and along the same lines of professional demarcation as those of the present. However, recent developments such as the extension of specialist roles for nurses, therapists and other healthcare professionals, and the rethinking of roles around an assessment of care pathways, are beginning to challenge these assumptions. The Government has encouraged the establishment of Workforce Development Confederations. These are intended to bring together employers, educators and professionals to plan the health service workforce and to look across different professional groups and the range of organisations that employ healthcare workers. A range of other measures designed to encourange and promote greater flexiblity in the workforce, are also being introduced, including reform of the pay system, a new Skills Escalator and the NHS University (NHSU).

However, the papers in this pamphlet suggest a much bolder approach is needed if the future health workforce is to deliver genuinely patient-centred care. They encourage us to recognise that communities and citizens, not just patients, have health needs that cannot be defined on the basis of clinical diagnosis alone but must instead reflect the importance of a far wider range of factors. So Stephen Fishwick and Melinda Letts suggest that performance targets and resources must reward attempts to improve people's quality of life and to increase levels of patient involvement, rather than focusing predominantly on activity rates in secondary care. Barbara Vaughan argues a more fundamental cultural shift is required, one that: 'moves away from the traditional paradigm from which healthcare has been developed to a broader based model, built on a mix of health and social well being.'

Achieving such a shift presents major challenges to the way that professional roles have traditionally been allocated and developed. Jeremy Wyatt and Cecilia Pyper both suggest that the types of practitioners required to meet new information needs and to provide care in new ways through ICT do not exist within the current workforce. Andrew Murdock and Barbara Vaughan, on the other hand, suggest that the skills that are needed in order to meet patients needs in relation to pharmacy and intermediate care are to be found amongst current practitioners. In the case of the intermediate care practitioner, the necessary skills are spread between different professionals and, in the case of the community pharmacist, they are embedded in a single professional role. However, Vaughan's analysis applies equally to both situations. She argues that:

> It is no longer viable or acceptable for each occupational group within the traditional team to

retain control over the aspects of work that have become the province of that group … In practice there are very few tasks that are limited to occupational groups since the essence of professional practice should be based on knowledge and judgement, neither of which can be monopolised by a single group.

The papers focusing on the development of the 'knowledge broker' and 'lay practitioner' indicate that the shift in roles and responsibilities that will be necessary in future will have a major imact on patients as well as health professionals.

The emerging issue for policy-makers is that broad changes in the way funding for patients is allocated and the way needs are assessed, could create much greater scope for innovation in the development of new roles. This will have implications for training and education, regulation and remuneration of healthcare workers. Both Andrew Murdoch and Barbara Vaughan suggest that in order to develop new practitioners, skills and competences will need to be more effectively shared across traditional professional boundaries. Finding different points of entry into the professions and 'crediting in' people who have relevant experience could help improve relationships between different professional groups. Wyatt, Pyper, and Fishwick and Letts all suggest new skills that could be developed amongst the existing workforce.

These papers have been written against a backdrop of a considerable re-examination of professional roles, brought about both by a government intent on reform and by a workforce under severe strain from staff shortages and the introduction of EU regulations to limit working hours. The impetus to seek imaginative solutions could not be greater. We hope this report provides a useful stimulus for future debate.

References

Kendall L (2001) *The Future Patient* London: ippr

Department of Health (2000) *The NHS Plan: A Plan for Investment. A Plan for Reform* London: TSO

Whittington Z et al. (2001) *Care at the Chemist: A Question of Access. A feasibility study comparing community pharmacy and general practice management of minor ailments* Report for the Community Pharmacy Research Consortium

Cabinet Office (2000) *Open all hours?* Results from the People's Panel, Issue 5

Audit Commission (2002) *A Focus on General Practice in England* London: Audit Commission

Exley S and Jarvis L (2001) *Trends in Attitudes to Health Care 1983 – 2000. Report based on results from the British Social Attitudes Surveys* National Centre for Social Research

2. The Consultant Pharmacist and Pharmacist Technician in Primary Care

Andrew Murdock

Executive summary

The NHS is currently in the process of rapid change and major structural reform. Consequently, those who practice within the NHS and those who interact with patients and professionals are questioning their working practices. This paper explores and proposes a new division of labour in community pharmacy that could allow pharmacists to maximise their contribution to patient care and help to relieve current pressures on the sector that is currently being experienced as a result of rising prescription volumes and workforce shortages. It highlights pharmacy's sporadic inclusion in expanding government policy and challenges current funding arrangements for the profession.

Introduction

Successive governments have acknowledged that pharmacists are an under-utilised resource within the NHS. The case for developing community pharmacy services has been discussed in policy documents from government and from the profession going back to the Nuffield report on Pharmacy in 1986 (Nuffield Foundation, 1986). Recently, however, policy makers have begun to take decisive steps towards enabling pharmacists to utilise and to build their skills through. Pharmacists are now playing an active role in co-ordinated self-care, prevention and early detection programmes, advice and awareness campaigns, formulary development and advising on rational, safe prescribing policies.

These actions chime with the need to make the best possible use of human resources. Evidence has suggested that pharmacists can reduce the burden of minor injuries as a proportion of GPs' workload by taking on responsibility for management of a range of minor injuries (Hassell *et al*, 2001). The recent extension of prescribing rights means that, by 2003, pharmacists will be able to prescribe a wider range of medicines on the basis of guidelines developed in conjunction with doctors and, more importantly, they will have a greater input into the monitoring of patient treatment plans. This extension of prescribing rights is expected to save around 2.5 million GP appointments for the treatment of minor injuries and ailments.

At a time when GP numbers and morale are at low ebb, evidence suggests that an enhanced role for pharmacists in repeat dispensing could also help to reduce GPs' workload. A recent report from the Regulatory Impact Unit has identified that nearly 2.75 million hours could be saved if pharmacists were to control the process of dispensing by instalments prescriptions written by a GP for a long term medical condition (Department of Health 2002).

Developing the role of community pharmacists will be a crucial element of implementing the public health agenda. The Government's aim of giving greater prominence to public health within the structures of the new NHS should involve, amongst other measures, utilisation of pooled budgets and integrated management structures across Primary Care Trusts and Local Authorities. Pharmacy, with its unique place at the heart of the community can become linked into the task of health promotion and disease prevention, acting as a sign-posting organisation and becoming a vital link between elements of the health service for patients.

However, bringing about these role changes whilst still providing the essential core dispensing service in a safe and efficient way, will require logistical, personnel and monetary re-engineering. At the moment insufficient remuneration, staff shortages and the absence of locum cover are among the reasons cited by pharmacists as barriers to their adoption of enhanced roles (Ruston, 2001). Re-allocating work from one healthcare professional's area to another without addressing resource issues for those taking on new roles only presents half a solution. Over the next five years the volume of prescriptions is set to rise by 33 percent, driven in part by the introduction of National Service Frameworks. From pharmacy's perspective, dealing with this spiralling increase in the volume of prescriptions whilst attempting to take on an extended role presents a significant logistical challenge.

Bold claims may be made about the ability of pharmacists to take on new roles but capacity within the pharmacy workforce can not be assumed. The 'fallow year' (when the pharmacy undergraduate course was extended from 3 to 4 years) has inevitably had an impact on pharmacist availability with virtually no pharmacists qualifying in 2001. The workforce across all of the pharmacy sectors is stretched. Government models predicted a 12% increase in demand between 1998-2003 for the private and NHS pharmacy workforce. Between 1993 and 2000 the number of students starting training increased by 27 per cent but still the problem is acute.

An ambitious vision of the pharmacist of the future is emerging and the opportunity should be taken. However, if limitations in pharmacists' capacity are to be met, bold and potentially controversial ideas about the division of labour and configuration of the pharmacy workforce must be considered. The following sections present for debate one vision of the way in which re-configuration of the role of community pharmacists could bring efficiency to the dispensing process and could allow expert pharmacists to maximise their contribution to the health service.

New pharmacy practitioners

If the full potential of pharmacy is to be recognised the current role of the pharmacist must be cleaved.

Certain responsibilities must be re-distributed amongst other members of the pharmacy team, namely the pharmacy technician team. This will create the critical time and space for the development of a Consultant Pharmacist with increasing clinical knowledge to interact productively with patients. Below these roles are outlined.

Consultant pharmacist

If we accept that GPs skills are primarily in diagnosis whilst pharmacists' skills centre on drug knowledge, the logical conclusion is that, in the fullness of time, GP prescriptions should detail a diagnosis with the decision making on the appropriate therapy becoming the responsibility of the pharmacist. This decision-making process is likely to include or require initial genetic testing to ascertain the suitability of certain drugs for patient enzyme systems. As we become increasingly aware of the interplay between drugs and body systems, it will become both easier and more important to monitor for possible adverse re-actions and this may well form an element of the pharmacists' role.

Pharmacists will also co-ordinate the dispensing process. Currently, patients or their carers either collect prescriptions from the surgery and take to the pharmacy for dispensing, or authorise a pharmacy to collect the prescriptions on their behalf and then either collect the prescription or have it delivered. Either way there is a patient journey required or reduced contact occurs between the patient and pharmacy staff. This does not always provide for optimal treatment and care.

With pharmacy controlling the repeat dispensing process, patients can be called to the pharmacy at appropriate intervals to have their health status checked rather than receiving, for example, a home delivery. This type of more frequent monitoring will detect inappropriate drug therapy or poor compliance sooner rather than later. Regular, closer scrutiny and involvement by the pharmacist will ensure that concordance can be reaffirmed which should again re-enforce better treatment outcomes to the benefit of all: patient, healthcare professionals and government. A patient being treated for hypertension, for example, could be asked to come to the pharmacy, or possibly even the pharmacist to visit them every third repeat prescription in order for the blood pressure to be measured. With the aid of technology the pharmacist could even provide patients with their own electronic sphygmomanometer, which can transmit readings down the telephone, for ratification.

With pharmacist prescriber status in place, modifications to treatment within the agreed patient plan or following nationally agreed protocols, will again produce better outcomes, better speed of response and thus greater patient satisfaction.

This combination of flexibility and prescribing status will allow community pharmacy handling of routine drug monitoring clinics. Traditionally these are carried out at a hospital outpatient clinic which may be time consuming and inconvenient for the patient. Delivery of this service at a local level close to the patient's home would be more cost-effective and less disruptive to the patient.

Expansion of the screening process to identify what we know are hugely under-diagnosed clinical conditions with a health time-bomb element attached to them is a natural extension of the process. For example in diabetes and hypertension we know that the potential secondary care complications manifested by not diagnosing the conditions early are great.

Pharmacy technician team

In essence, then, the routine dispensing function will be a process delegated to skilled dispensers with input from the pharmacist still maintained where appropriate. The dispensing process will be further augmented with the use of 'automats' (automated dispensing systems) facilitated by computerised workflow management systems.

In addition, there will be greater use of accredited checking technicians (a role more commonly found in the hospital sector but beginning to develop within the community arena). These technicians are trained to oversee and approve, within agreed guidelines, the mechanical aspect of the dispensing process. There is also absolutely no reason why a higher-grade technician should not be established, say a dispensary manager, responsible for all dispensary activity. It must be made clear from the outset that skilled pharmaceutical assessment of prescriptions, will still require pharmacist clearance.

Practice location

The measures proposed above are focused primarily on pharmacists working at a primary care level. Indeed, this is where the thrust of future treatment should be. However, this still leaves open the question of the most effective delivery point for pharmacy. Some will argue that it should be purely from within the domain of a health centre or 'One-Stop' Primary Care Centre. There is logic to this: it is valid to suggest that the degree of interactivity required between the myriad of healthcare professionals can only take place with professionals working within the same premises. Yet this risks ignoring a primary dynamic: that healthcare should be delivered as close to the patient's community as possible. Thus whilst one might expect a natural preponderance of the concept within the 'One-Stop Family' this would not be the only delivery mechanic: heavy 'community pharmacy' engagement from 'traditional' community locations should also be expected.

If patient care is to become seamless, the primary/secondary care front will require examination and refinement. The removal of outpatient dispensing duties from the hospital sector to primary care will allow more crucial clinical time for hospital pharmacists. Efficiency will be increased still further if the pharmaceutical aspects of hospital pre-admission are dealt with in the community where there is a more complete knowledge of patient medication, including drugs purchased for self-care.

The development of these roles, however, relies on developments in other policy areas. Widening the prescribing gateway, for example, depends on significant improvements in communication and record keeping. Pharmacists' integration into the primary health team is contingent on the development of Electronic Transfer of Prescriptions and the introduction of a common health record. The Government's wishes in this respect have been communicated in recent publications (Department of Health, 2002) and rejuvenated by the Treasury's Wanless Report (Wanless, 2002). Yet many within the profession are sceptical about the pace of progress. In the past, one of the factors limiting pharmacists from development of their role has been continuing refusal for connectivity to NHSnet. Pharmacists must be included within an integrated IT system if hopes for their future role are to be realised. Assigning of a specific-healthcare professional be it dentist, doctor, optician or pharmacist to a patient ensures identified professional accountability and a treatment continuum. To achieve this, will require patient registration with a number of healthcare professionals delivering slightly different services.

Policy implications

This separation and redefinition of roles within pharmacy requires an educational rethink. In essence what is proposed is the formation of a two-tier pharmacy qualification: a dispensing pharmacist, whose responsibilities extend no further than that process and a consultant pharmacist who would engage in the diagnostic testing, medicine management and more extended role aspects of the profession, but in all cases linked to the supply function.

Suggestions of deviation from today's current pharmacy practice will provoke responses ranging from nervousness to heresy. The creation of a two-tier pharmacist system coupled with delegating aspects of the work, seen by many as the crux of today's operation, will attract numerous critics. Considerable effort, debate and discussion will be required to persuade the profession that this is the correct course of action and strong professional leadership will be required. However, the march of technology, coupled with the valuable opportunity for moving closer to realising the pharmacist's contribution to patient-care, demand a radical rethink of this nature.

Realignment of the profession provides challenges for both training and regulation:

Training

Currently the single pharmacy qualification requires a 4-year university course followed by a pre-registration year with a concluding exam before a pharmacist may practice. Dispensing technician qualifications are either by an NVQ or a BTech route. The current system is inflexible in allowing crossover from technician to pharmacist: a technician who aspires to become a qualified dispensing pharmacist would have to start from the beginning of the university training process, without any recourse made to any technician qualification that they may currently hold.

The expanding pharmaceutical qualification poses a question on expanding the entry points into the profession. Capability should be made to allow those with other or partial health related qualifications to be given credits that could be offset against the degree courses rather than a mature student having to start from base-level. This again will require creativity from the universities and the professional body. The course re-structuring opportunity should also allow greater inclusion of social factors and the re-engineering of teaching into case studies, which would incorporate all aspects of pharmaceutical knowledge, rather than the silo process that still occurs today. It would be more meaningful and aspects of pharmacy taught today, which in isolation could be questioned for their relevance, would be put into perspective.

The role of the 'consultant pharmacist' would be achieved by building on the current qualification with competency-based assessment. This could start to deliver some of the roles outlined in *Pharmacy in the Future*. In turn this would then aid PCTs in delivering not only the national but also their local targets.

Registration

The creation of the 'dispensing pharmacist' grade would under clinical governance aspirations require registration, as would some of the higher technician grades. This will require the profession to identify the appropriate registration body. This has already initiated some heated debate. Currently only pharmacists are registered with the Royal Pharmaceutical Society, although the latter, along with the Health Professions Council, are logical choices for the registration of technicians.

Representation

However, the development of new roles for pharmacists can not be considered in isolation from other measures necessary if they are to play a more active part within the primary care team. To ensure the existence of uniform planning across the health and social professions there must also be appropriate representation of the professions on primary care boards and at executive level. This has so far been steadfastly refused in England but not so in Wales where there is a more all embracing and sensible approach.

Recent indications from the first wave of NHS LIFT projects also appear to identify a lack of total inclusion. NHS LIFT is a joint venture scheme for the redevelopment of the primary care estate. The whole raison d'être of LIFT is to ensure that future health needs of the community are taken into account so that the 'bricks and mortar' can be designed and placed accordingly. However, there is some evidence to suggest that, from a community pharmacy perspective, this has not occurred. If integrated planning cannot be achieved there is little hope in achieving government aspirations. Pharmacy, and community pharmacy in particular, allows easy access to healthcare. Government should bear this in mind in future planning and avoid the debacle that occurred when pharmacy had to fight its corner vigorously to be included in the referral algorithms for NHS Direct.

Remuneration

Pharmacy's current remuneration and reimbursement formulae are now outmoded and require revisiting. The existing system does not reward or encourage effective healthcare, it only provides for the physical dispensing of prescriptions. Even then there is a mismatch between volumes processed and monies paid.

Whilst the ever-increasing devolution of budgets to PCTs provides for localised healthcare ownership, there is a danger that as a bi-product this could result in payment fragmentation and distorted rates for similar services across the country. The introduction of local pharmaceutical services could easily exacerbate the situation. This must be guarded against. It will become divisive and may do nothing for standards.

A holistic funding formula, which considers the dispensing, drug purchase element and the extended role is paramount. To determine this, some appreciation must be had of the cost of providing such a service. In that way a sensible rate of return for providers can be calculated.

Conclusion

If pharmacy is to realise its potential contribution to patient care, action is needed across a range of policy areas. This paper has suggested that a cleavage of the role of community pharmacists is required: allowing a Consultant Pharmacist to focus on decision making about therapies on the basis of diagnosis from the GP and relying on a well-trained pharmacy technician team to carry out the routine dispensing function. In order for these roles to be developed, the structure of professional qualifications must be reconsidered. Entry points into the profession need to be re-evaluated with greater flexibility being established between healthcare professional courses and technician courses to allow a degree of interchange. University courses need to be redesigned to allow teaching of the pharmacy course in a case study manner rather than subject silo mode.

The Government must make real its stated ambitions for pharmacy by ensuring that community pharmacists are genuinely included in the process of primary care services development. Schemes for the development of the primary care estate, such as NHS LIFT, should include all healthcare professionals in its planning to produce an accurate requirement for the distribution of health needs across the population and pharmacists must have places of right on PCT or, in future, Care Trust boards.

References

Department of Health (2000) *Pharmacy in the Future – Implementing the NHS Plan* London: TSO

Department of Health (2002) *Public Sector Making a Difference* Regulatory Impact Unit London: TSO

Department of Health (2002) *Delivering IT in the NHS – A Summary of the national programme for IT* London: TSO

Hassell K, Whittington Z, Cantrill J, Bates F, Rogers A and Noyce P (2001) *Care at the Chemist; A Question of Access – a feasibility study comparing community pharmacy and general practice management of minor ailments* Manchester: University of Manchester

Nuffield Foundation (1986) *Pharmacy: The report of a committee of inquiry* London: Nuffield Foundation

Ruston A (2001) 'Achieving re-professionalisation: factors that influence the adoption of an 'extended role' by community pharmacists' in *Journal of Social and Administrative Pharmacy* Vol 18 No 3 pp 103-110

Wanless D (2002) *Securing our Future Health: Taking a Long-Term View: Final Report* London: TSO

3. The Telecarer: a new role for clinical professionals

Professor Jeremy C. Wyatt

Executive summary

Health systems world-wide are subject to new drivers and opportunities for change. Many of these, including patients' desire for quick and easy access to healthcare, staff shortages and a continued drive towards cost-efficiency, contribute towards the emergence of various new health professional roles. This paper outlines a specific new role, already being pioneered by the 700 nurses working in NHS Direct call centres who use the phone to triage, inform and counsel seven million callers per year. We call this role a telecarer: a health professional who delivers services and support to remote patients or clients using the most appropriate communications media such as telephone, email or digital TV.

Introduction

A telecarer is a health professional who delivers responsive, high quality services and support to remote patients or clients using the most appropriate and accepted communications media, colleagues and information sources. Four key drivers are contributing to the emergence of this new telecarer role: technology, patient demand, healthcare workforce pressures and health service policies.

Technology

Two kinds of technological development favour the emergence of telecare and the telecarer. The first is improved sensor technology which includes low cost, portable or even implanted sensors and disposable testing kits to assist home-based clinical measurement in chronic diseases, such as blood glucose for diabetes, peak flow rate for asthma or weight, blood pressure and cholesterol for coronary artery disease. A new development is the ability to directly download data from these sensors to a web-based virtual patient record or whole life 'health biography' for charting on screen, or even to drive decision support systems (Peckham, 2000).

The second is advances in Information and Communications Technology (ICT). A wide range of cheaper 'information appliances' such as the cell phone, interactive digital TV (iDTV) or radio-linked personal data assistants (PDAs) integrated into cell phones are becoming available. Technology has also reduced the costs of always-on Internet connections, providing a sustainable model for telecare and the intensive monitoring needed for hospital at home projects.

Patient demand

Patients' increasing use of NHS and private walk-in centres and NHSDirect phone and online services indicate that a health system must adapt to the public's desire to access the health information or service they want, when they want it, through the most convenient medium. Telecare could offer a further response to the problems patients identify with the current health system such as poor co-ordination of care across the primary-secondary care divide and unequal distribution of services or access to expertise (BMA, 2000).

A greater use of telecare has the potential to make particular impact on care of the growing proportion of patients with chronic diseases. As HMOs in the USA have shown, improving the quality of care for patients with chronic diseases mean frequent brief contacts, not occasional treks to a hospital outpatient department. Telecare will also make it easier to involve as 'expert patient' advocates in the community who lack the resources to travel to and participate in face to face clinical encounters. Given that patients forget much of what they are told in hospital outpatient departments, it seems likely they will welcome advice sent by email or shared electronically with a relative, even hundreds of miles away.

Healthcare workforce pressures

The NHS is chronically short of skilled staff with, for example, half the mean EU number of doctors per 1000 population (OECD, 2001). Initiatives to increase staff numbers are in the pipeline but the EU Working Time Directive and inevitable delays in attaining staffing targets mean that measures to find more efficient ways of working will be necessary. Aside from staff shortages there are other, positive, pressures from the healthcare workforce that might contribute towards the development of the telecarer role. Telecaring, in offering the possibility of home-based working, could represent one way of meeting the desire for flexible working, career breaks and increasing proportions of women medical students. Telecaring could also make it easier for professionals to share their summary of a patient's problem and agreed plan with a more dispersed team of colleagues and patient relatives. Also, electronic logging of professional activity and support from remote peers will aid life-long learning and help professionals to assemble their portfolio for revalidation.

Health service policies

Telecaring is a tool to facilitate a number of broad NHS and related policy goals. There are, for example, public and policy pressures to create services that promote independence and enable patients to remain at home where possible, in order to reduce risks of cross-infection, encourage self care and to respond to patients' desire to avoid hospital stays where possible. This is leading to the growth of day surgery and other forms of day care. Telecare will complement these models and may make these forms of service provision safer and more viable.

Where telecaring is adopted it should be as part of the process, used in National Service Frameworks, of developing systems around an assessment of patient need. Its potential is enhanced by current policy moves towards expanding nurse's role through prescribing and the use of protocols. This practice has recently been strengthened by systematic review evidence that primary care nurse practitioners are as effective as doctors and better accepted by patients (Horrocks, 2002) and suggestions that less senior staff are often better at following guidelines and applying organisational solutions (Wyatt, 2001).

Adoption of the telecarer role could form part of the eGov targets to increase the proportion of citizen-government communications made using electronic media and complement NHS Information strategies. These emphasise network and encryption infrastructure for NHS staff and organisations, computer based prescribing and a virtual electronic health record infrastructure (DoH, 1998; 2001; 2002). Taken together, these pressures and policy drivers will lead to the emergence of telecaring as a significant part of the working life of most health professionals.

Outline of the telecarer role

Over the next five years, more and more people who are sick or worried about their health will communicate with the health system by phone and by email, SMS message, interactive digital TV, radio-linked personal data assistants or web-linked clinical measurement devices from their own home, work or other sites. Some communication needs will be met by automatic systems (for example, through browsing NHSDirect online). But there will be many cases where the person seeks human reassurance, is unable or unwilling to navigate electronic information resources or wants advice or other services specifically tailored to their needs. These people will still require a human response.

Patient-professional email consultation is still relatively uncommon in the UK but is a far more convenient and enduring medium that the telephone. In a study of patient use of email to doctors in the US four years ago, each email took the doctor about four minutes to read and answer (Borowitz, 1998). So ten patient emails a day would demand an extra four hours per week of each GP or nurse practitioner's time (equivalent to an extra session for GPs).

Of course, the many face-to-face contacts about health matters with GPs, nurses, retail pharmacists and other health professionals in primary care and A&E will continue. However, an increase in new forms of communication means that the NHS must create and train a new cadre of telecarers: health professionals who can use these new media to fluently communicate with patients and the public about health matters. Like the NHSDirect nurses who continue to work part time in A&E departments, many of these telecarers will be existing professionals spending some of their week working in this new role.

Figure 3.1: The role of the telecarer, mediating between patients in the community and the physical NHS

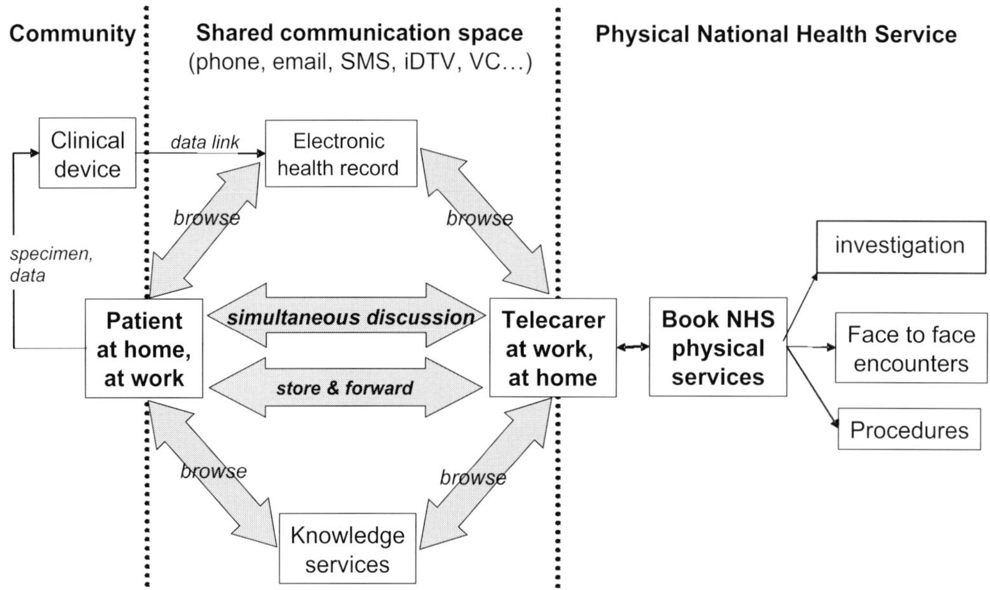

The role of a telecarer shown in Figure 3.1 will include both technical and communication aspects. The main technical roles will be:

- becoming fluent with setting up and using their selected media for communicating with patients and the public, to the extent that they can help patients improve their own use of that medium;
- knowing what can be safely communicated over the medium, and about inherent problems such as delayed response times or loss of privacy;
- being familiar with how to maximise the effectiveness of the medium, for exmaple, requesting a photo of a skin ulcer attached to an email, if the patient has a digital camera at home

The main human and communication roles will be:

- learning how to build sustainable patient relationships over the medium without eroding patient trust in their face-to-face health provider;
- knowing what patient support resources are available on that medium and being able to direct patients to them; some telecarers will develop their own patient support resources;
- being able to document a consultation and the information given to a patient in the electronic health record so that other health providers are aware of the contact and its content.

A telecarer could be a specialist in their own right (a cyber doctor or nurse) or telecaring could be a significant activity of generalists or specialists. Some specialists are already part-time telecarers, for example doctors participating in teledermatology or telepsychiatry sessions. However, unlike NHSDirect nurses, these doctors receive hardly any training to support this major change in their working practices. The Foresight report (Peckham, 2000), predicts that by 2015 people will be interacting with a 'cyber physician' by using voice recognition, a web-held patient biography and an interactive TV wall. All this technology is available now, so by 2015 a virtual or automaton telecarer could be an economically attractive front end to health services. To illustrate the telecarer role it is useful here to explore a near-future scenario in which a nurse telecarer Sally manages an unstable diabetic, Mrs Patel.

A Hypothetical Telecare Interaction

Mrs Patel, a 27 year old solicitor, has diabetes controlled on insulin 20 units per day. She measures her blood sugar daily using a device that sends results to her own password-protected NHS diabetes web page. Sally, the general practice telecare nurse, works from home most days and regularly checks Mrs Patel's web page, emailing her to attend the surgery for a glycosylated haemoglobin (HbA1C) test when needed.

Last Monday, Sally noticed that Mrs Patel's blood sugar was high three times over the weekend. The diabetes NSF suggests an HbA1C today followed by review of insulin dose. At 10am, Sally sends Mrs Patel an email with automatic reading notification. However, by 3pm the email has still not been read. Sally sends an SMS message to Mrs Patel's mobile, another email and one to Mr Patel, whose e-ddress she finds through a web-based address book. She also posts an urgent message on Mrs Patel's personal web page with instructions to attend for the blood test then hands over Mrs Patel's details to the regional diabetic telecare centre and goes off duty. About 5pm Mrs Patel's meeting finishes so she turns on her mobile and receives the SMS message and logs onto her web page. Using the information posted by Sally, she attends for the blood test on her way home. The result is posted on her personal web page by 7pm, together with a link to the relevant section of the NSF protocol with a suggestion that Mrs Patel calls Sally tomorrow for a chat. The next day Mrs Patel checks the NSF protocol for her new insulin dose. Sally calls and books an urgent virtual meeting with a diabetology telecarer using his online diary.

The virtual review meeting takes place on Tuesday afternoon with Mrs Patel, Sally and Dr Jones contributing comments as and when they can over a couple of hours during other duties, using Mrs Patel's web page as a shared discussion space. During the meeting Mrs Patel reveals that she missed a period 6 weeks ago and had a positive pregnancy test last Friday. Sally and Dr Jones agree she should increase her regular insulin to 24 units, fix a further follow up in 2 weeks (setting automatic reminders in their online diaries) and exchange notes about which NSF sections are most helpful at this early stage of pregnancy.

This short scenario illustrates the various roles of the telecarer and the need for them to be fluent in using the following media and services for communicating patient data and accessing medical knowledge:

- telephone, voicemail and SMS messaging
- email with automatic notification of reading
- data downloaded automatically from a device to a web site
- password protected web pages and web forms
- web-mediated discussion session

- online address books, diaries and setting automated reminders

This leads to the draft specification, see box 3.1

Box 3.1: Draft person specification for a telecarer

- An experienced clinical gatekeeper with wide knowledge of the NHS, social and other services
- Clinical expertise specific to a chronic disease or problem, or wider clinical skills such as primary care triage
- Excellent communication skills and ability to establish rapport over various communication media, especially with patients and carers
- Excellent familiarity with a critical mass of current media (telephone, GSM mobile, email, web, videoconferencing, iDTV…) and services (voicemail, SMS, conference calls, virtual discussion sessions, online address books, online diaries, risk calculators, interactive disease management protocols…)

Optional:

- the ability to set up or revise the content of voicemail and telephone menu systems, web sites, etc.
- An ability to work consistently unsupervised, excellent personal organisational skills
- An ability to recognise typical clinical problems and find, adapt and apply NHS-mandated solutions, rather than always inventing their own solution (Wyatt, 2001)

Policy implications of the telecarer role

To develop and deliver this telecarer role fully within the NHS will require the collection of an evidence base about the types of telecarer interventions that are popular, safe and cost effective. It raises a number of problems and will require several changes to, or developments of, existing policies.

Developing the evidence base

In order for telecaring to be pursued, there must be evidence to suggest that it contributes towards improvements in outcomes, is appreciated by patients as well and is safe and cost-effective.

So far, the evidence about patient attitudes towards new ways of communicating with health professionals is inconclusive. A systematic review of patient satisfaction with telemedicine reveals some evidence that patients are willing to participate in telecare (Mair, 2000). However the studies of real time video consultations reviewed were found to be of variable quality and limited generalisability.

They illustrated that patients, for the most part, found teleconsultation acceptable. Some patients appreciated increased ease of access to experts, reduced travel or waiting times. However, others worried about the worsened quality of communication with the remote expert.

The question of whether telecare and telemedicine actually improve the quality of care and patient outcomes is critical. A Cochrane systematic review identified 7 Randomised Control Trials studying a total of 800 people (Currell, 2000). In all studies the technology was reliable. In one study patient acceptance was good and in the only other study in which acceptance was evaluated it was neutral. In one study of virtual outreach, study patients spent only half an hour at a GP surgery compared to 2.5hrs in hospital for control patients. Five trials measured patient outcomes, but only one of these was positive, with improved medication adherence and a bigger drop in diastolic BP.

There is also systematic review evidence that 'distance medicine' (mainly telephone communication between patients and health staff) improves clinical practice in 78 per cent of 97 comparisons and patient outcomes in 78 per cent of 27 comparisons (Balas, 1998): see Box 3.2. However, despite some significant savings, the review showed insufficient evidence of cost-effectiveness.

Box 3.2: Randomised trial evidence of improvement in clinical practice or patient outcome from 'distance medicine'

Health workers using phone / network to contact patients: 66 RCTs

Patients or carers contacting health system: 14 RCTs

Huge range of technology, purposes, diseases and outcome measures studied

Positive outcomes or improved performance:

- Computerised communication (modem / phone data transfer): 7 (100%) of 7 trials
- Interactive telephone menu system: 6 (83%) of 7 trials
- After hours telephone: 3 (75%) of 4 trials
- Telephone reminders: 14 (61%) of 23 trials
- Telephone follow-up & counseling: 20 (54%) of 37 trials
- Telephone screening: 1 (33%) of 3 trials

(adapted from Balas, 1998)

The lack of an evidence base for the cost-effectiveness of telecare must be addressed in order for the telecarer role to be fully developed. However, it is still worthwhile considering the further implications of the role, given that these practitioners already exist and are likely to grow in number, evidence or no evidence.

Education, training and validation of telecarers and clinical professionals

With rapid changes in communications technology and the potential risks associated with remote care, it is important for potential telecarers to participate in a training course and obtain a telecaring certificate to complement their clinical training. If and when telecaring starts to form a significant part of the role of most health professionals, such courses will become a routine component of continuing professional development and then undergraduate courses.

Adequate knowledge of and skills in telecare, participation in such courses and evidence of telecarer experience could be conditions attached to professional validation and revalidation. One problem for full-time telecarers will be fewer opportunities for learning direct from other clinical professionals. Although e-learning is an obvious possibility and is being developed by the NHS University, some telecarers will already be spending most of their working life communicating by phone or the internet. Thus, it might be better for them to rotate through real clinical posts weekly or monthly.

Privacy of data and authentication of telecarers and entitled citizens

There is already widespread concern over the privacy of sensitive patient data held on paper or electronic media, and with telecarers working from home using a variety of media to communicate with patients this could lead to further breaches of confidentiality. Some possible scenarios could include:

- a patient fails to clear medical data on web forms held in the browser cache on an internet café or shared work computer; friends or co-workers learn of their psychiatric problems;
- legitimate monitoring by employers of employee emails or web sites visited leads to realisation by manager that patient has epilepsy or HIV, who then discriminates against employee;
- the teenage son of a telecarer working from home gets access to emails from patients seeking advice on sexual matters, responds inappropriately using parent's log in;
- a mother curious about repeated calls on daughter's cell phone bill, dials a number that turns out to be the NHS teenage pregnancy help line;
- an unauthorised, unscrupulous life insurance executive employs a private detective to identify members of the public contacting an NHS Cancer help line.

With telecaring becoming more frequent, such potential threats to data privacy will become more complex to manage because patient data, including simple contact details, will spread outside the range of routine security precautions available within the NHS (for example, NHSNet firewalls), into the homes of telecarers and onto their notebook PCs or cell phones. Appropriate encryption and other precautions such as biometric identification of the device user will be necessary to prevent privacy lapses of the kinds described above.

A further potential difficulty is the need for authentication of both telecarers and patients. Few patients would be duped by a bogus health professional when they meet them face-to-face, but cyber doctors and other carers with fake or dubious qualifications are not unusual on the web (Eysenbach, 1998). Patients must be able to tell that their telecarer holds the claimed qualifications as well as a certificate of telecaring. In return, the telecarer needs to reliably identify the person they are communicating with, for two reasons. First, they need to add data to the correct electronic record, and prevent rare attempts by impostors to masquerade as the patient. Second, except in emergencies, telecarers must check that each client is entitled to NHS services (for example, that the email is not from someone with no NHS entitlement). This suggests the need for a central web-based register of both qualified telecarers and UK citizens.

Other informatics aspects of telecare

One major requirement of the telecarer is that they summarise each encounter and make it accessible to everyone managing the patient from the standard EHR interface, whatever medium the exchange took place in. NHSDirect keep a tape recording of the full caller transaction to answer patient enquiries and even later legal challenges. The NHS will need to provide this long term data storage since telecoms provider's archives are quite transient (for example: SMS messages are kept for only 3 months).

Turning to knowledge management, we will need to ensure that the same version of NHS reference material and guidelines are available to the public across all the communication media they choose to use. These should give advice compatible with that from NHS knowledge sources for professionals (Wyatt, 2001b).

To ensure that the service is truly inclusive, NHSNet and associated voice and other networks will need to be extended to include every UK home and workplace. It will also need to include mobile devices such as cell phones and wireless PDAs, and to certain classes of fixed or implanted clinical monitoring devices such as blood glucose, peak flow or activity sensors. Virtual private network (VPN) methods may be an appropriate model for this.

Quality assurance, patient safety, legal and management issues

Despite adequate training and certification of telecarers, things could go badly wrong for patients through telecarer illness, incompetence or even malicious acts without the awareness of professional peers. This is partly because the flexible staff working arrangements resulting from telecaring could bring with them isolation and fragmentation of the caring professions. This suggests a number of measures will be needed to ensure the quality of care, in addition to the training and certification already discussed.

Carefully written clinical guidelines or care pathways, like the ones developed for NHSDirect, will be necessary to ensure that telecarers apply proven solutions in which everyone understands their role and future plans. A chronic illness guideline might include an obligatory 3-monthly review by another telecarer. We know that patients greatly value continuity of provider, or at least that the next provider knows the key details of their problem (BMA, 2000). Telecarer managers will need to establish mechanisms for ensuring continuity and handover within defined teams with an ability to escalate or reduce the intensity of care being delivered according to patients' needs. There will also be a need for national standards for maximum response times and codes of practice to address unexpected absence of telecarers and guidelines on privacy issues. Some of these may be informed by a code of practice for doctor-patient email published by the American Medical Informatics Association (www.amia.org).

As a new model of care, telecaring raises some challenging legal liability issues. For example, will a court consider a telecarer an autonomous health professional? What happens if a telecarer expresses doubts about managing a patient through a narrow communication medium and requests a face-to-face appointment, but the patient does not arrive: is there then an obligation to visit the patient at home or contact a relative? Can the NHS refuse to telecare a patient with clinical monitors at home if the patient fails to take care of their monitors and communication links? Work on the legal issues around telemedicine (Stanberry, 1998) will illuminate some of these questions, but some will remain unanswered until actual court cases will provide clarification.

The growth in the number of telecarers will also raise management questions. For example, it is unclear to which part of the NHS telecarers will belong, and to whom they should report. Since they do not work only in primary, community or secondary care, perhaps a new NHS 'Cyber Care' Division will need to be created. Management methods and information systems will need to be developed to remotely monitor telecarer workload and divide incoming patient contacts, while maintaining continuity of care as much as possible. This will probably mean retaining some kind of geographical organisation, despite the temptation to organise all NHS telecarers by disease or clinical problem areas. For reasons of continuing professional development and quality improvement, virtual telecare centres with 50-150 home or mobile workers and a small physical base for administration and face-to-face meetings and training seem likely.

Access, equity, inclusiveness of the health system

There is rightly much concern over possible 'cyber-divides', including those who cannot pay hardware or telecoms charges and those who lack the skills or ability to learn how to use the internet or cell phones. Interactive digital TV (iDTV) is an easy to use, less flexible but more pervasive medium than internet-connected PCs. Over 97 per cent of homes currently have a TV and millions already have an iDTV; iDTV will become the only way to receive broadcast TV in the UK by 2006. Telecarer and other services designed for iDTV and other media will need to respect the reduced sensory abilities of the elderly and those with chronic illness, as well as those whose first language is not English. There are already 45 million cell phones in the UK including pre pay phones used by children and young people, so message or voice communication with telecarers should be possible with most who wish it.

However, a firm and enduring principle of the NHS is that access is free at point of care delivery. Telecare is a new form of care delivery and must also be free at the point of care. With each call to

NHSDirect lasting 10-20 minutes, a free phone number could add to £10m to their annual operating cost, so they opted for an 0845 local rate number. However, this may still deter some callers. Thus, we will need to provide new forms of NHS free phone, 'free text' or 'free net' access points; this would be much simpler than reimbursing patients for using telecoms services to contact the NHS.

Obstacles or threats to the growth of telecaring

We must also consider potential threats to the adoption and growth of telecare and telecarers. These fit under three headings: failure of the public to use advanced technology, professional barriers and organisational problems such as insufficient investment in ICT.

Failure of the public to use advanced technology

The need for public support for telecare has already been stated. An unlikely but possible future position, perhaps precipitated by media frenzy over a series of telecaring accidents, could be extreme popular scepticism about such technology: the 'wood world' scenario described in our Foresight report (Peckham, 2000). The public reaction to GMO based food is an instructive example of how popular anti-science reactions may be stoked by the media; the solution is careful examination of the evidence on effectiveness, and listening to the views of the public during pilot studies.

A further an important concern is the 'cyberdivide', with internet access available to or used by only a small proportion of those who need access to telecarers. We know there is lingering public scepticism about the internet. For example, a recent Consumer's Association survey showed that a quarter of the UK population have no plans to go online because of high costs or perceived irrelevance to them (Consumer Association, 2002).

Professional barriers

Poor preparation and training of health professionals together with conservative or protectionist professional organisations, fearful of a perceived threat to their identity or power, might lead to reluctance or even refusal to adopt the telecaring model of healthcare. This is especially likely if telecaring becomes an additional responsibility, instead of substituting for some face-to-face clinical activities.

Organisational barriers

There are two main uncertainties here. First, insufficient investment in ICT to support adequate infrastructure or the reimbursement of telecoms charges would clearly slow development of this role. Second, continuing uncertainty over the quality of care delivered by telecarers or doubts over their legal status, and that of the organisations who train and employ them, could lead to slow uptake of this new model of care.

Conclusions

A key question is: how to start? The answer seems to be to build on existing services such as extending the NHSDirect telephone help line or the promised email enquiry service for NHSDirect Online to chronic disease management. Once these are up and running, evaluation can be carried out to examine safety, cost and efficacy issues. Further clinical niches could be added where most relevant, such as post hospital discharge, or follow up after starting any new therapy. Clearly the barriers listed above need to be addressed where possible and pilots should be evaluated to make sure that both positive and negative lessons are learned and disseminated.

Overall, we see the emergence of the telecarer role in the work of more and more health professionals over the next three to five years as inevitable, but support and training and actions to resolve the quality and information issues described above will be essential.

Acknowledgements: With thanks to Sylvia Wyatt and Justin Keen for comments and support

References

Balas E, Jaffrey F, Kuperman GJ, Boren SA, Brown GD, Pinciroli F and Mitchell J (1997) 'Electronic communication with patients - evaluation of distance medicine technology' in *Journal of the American Medical Association* (JAMA); 278: 152-9

BMA Policy Unit (2000) 'Literature review: what sort of healthcare do the public expect, want or need?' in *Healthcare Funding Review* Annex 1. London: BMA

Borowitz S and Wyatt J (1998) 'The origin, content and workload of electronic mail consultation' in *Journal of the American Medical Association* (JAMA) 280: 1321-4

Consumer Society Survey 2002 published on the BBC website http://news.bbc.co.uk/1/hi/uk/827706.stm

Currell R, Urquhart C, Wainwright P and Lewis R (2000). Telemedicine versus face to face patient care: effects on professional practice and healthcare outcomes. Cochrane Database Syst Rev 2000;(2):CD002098

Eysenbach G and Diepgen TL (1998) 'Responses to unsolicited patient email requests for medical advice on the World Wide Web' in *Journal of the American Medical Association* (JAMA); 280: 1333-5

Horrocks S, Anderson E and Salisbury C (2002) 'Systematic review of whether nurse practitioners working in primary care can provide equivalent care to doctors' *BMJ*; 324: 819-23

Horton R (2002) 'Nurse-prescribing in the UK: right but also wrong' *Lancet*; 359: 1875-6

Mair F and Whitten P. (2000) 'Systematic review of studies of patient satisfaction with telemedicine' *BMJ*; 320: 1517-20

OECD (2001) Health Data 2001

Peckham M (Chair, Foresight healthcare panel) (2000) *Heathcare 2020* Department for Trade and Industry, Foresight 2000. www.foresight.gov.uk

Stanberry BA (1998) *The legal & ethical aspects on telemedicine* London: Royal Society of Medicine Press

Wyatt JC (2001a) *Clinical knowledge and practice in the information age: a handbook for health professionals* RSM Press

Wyatt JC (2001b) 'Knowledge for the Clinician 10. Management of explicit and tacit knowledge' *Journal of the Royal Society of Medicine* 94: 6-9

4. The Public Health Leader

by Ruth Tennant and David Woodhead

Executive summary

The determinants of health are complex. biological, social and economic factors all have strong and overlapping effects. Similarly, the responses needed to improve health need to be multifaceted and cover a range of medical, social and economic policy areas. Effective interventions act at international, national and local levels and take multi-sectoral approaches. Concerted action in single areas will not yield long term, sustainable results.

The public health workers of the future will increasingly reflect the need for comprehensive and cross-sectoral approaches, breaking from the biomedical dominance of the past. The agenda has now broadened and those working in public health in the future will come from a wide variety of backgrounds and perspectives too numerous to list here. They might be medically trained or come from a community development background. They might be trained in environmental health or housing, or in health visiting or health promotion. They will work in networks where the part each different practitioner plays will be recognised and systems will ensure co-ordination of their action. Co-ordination requires strong leadership, which will be provided practitioners who are able to work across a range of agencies, bringing together diverse practitioners to deliver on public health objectives. This paper explores the role of these Public Health Leaders of the future and the policies necessary to ensure success.

Introduction

Public health may lack some of the perceived glamour of hospital-based medicine. However, since 1854 when John Snow worked out that victims of a cholera outbreak on Broad Street in Soho could be traced back to a single water pump, public health has been at the centre of measures to prevent illness and improve population health. Over the last few years, there has been increasing debate around the precise role and purpose of the public health function – and the precise role of public health workers. Simultaneously, there has been a growing recognition that the medical model of public health, with its emphasis on the prevention of specific diseases through screening, immunisation and disease control is just one part of a wider public health function that needs to act upon the broader determinants of health.

The 1998 Independent Inquiry into Inequalities in Health (Acheson, 1998) helped advance this argument by reinforcing the case made 20 years earlier in the Black Report (Black, 1980) that factors including (but not limited to) unemployment, poor education and poor quality housing had a major impact on health status. The Government's initial response to this was cautious with its public health

White Paper *Saving Lives: Our Healthier Nation* (Department of Health, 1999), which focused on disease-based targets for heart disease, stroke, cancer, mental health (suicides) and accidents. However, this White Paper was followed by the more ambitious introduction by the Treasury of 'national health inequalities targets' which require sustained, multi-sectoral input to achieve.

Although health improvement has become increasingly high profile, it is just one component of public health's wide remit. Responsibilities for communicable disease control and investigation, environmental health and contributing to emergency planning are central to the public health function. Concerns about biological and chemical incidents in the wake of the events of September 11th 2001 and a new strategy for infectious diseases (Chief Medical Officer 2001) have reinforced the need for strong leadership, effective delivery structures and adequate resources to support this component of the public health function.

However public health is already delivered through a wide variety of different staff. In addition to primary care trust-based public health teams nad new local health protection services a much range of staff inside the NHS, local government and voluntary sector, contribute towards meeting public health objectives. The new public health workforce will need to reflect the growing breadth and complexity of public health responsibilities. Delivering public health goals can only be achieved by a multi-skilled and multi-dimensional workforce including both medically and non-medically trained public health specialists, information analysts, health promotion experts, working closely with an even broader range of staff needed to deliver public health goals on the ground.

A number of new initiatives have been put in place to strengthen the public health function and to reflect its broad remit. Public health training schemes have been opened up to people without a previous medical qualification, opening up senior posts in public health to non-medics. As part of the 2002 NHS reorganisation, public health delivery has been moved closer to communities with the responsibility for delivering public health locally being devolved down to PCTs. Directors of Public Health now sit on all PCT boards and their input will be central to meeting PCTs' responsibilities to improve the health of the populations they serve. New public health networks, covering strategic health authority areas will pool specialist skills where it is not economical for each PCT to have these skills in-house.

Although these changes have been broadly welcomed by managers, specialists and practitioners working in public health (Woodhead *et al,* 2002) concerns have been raised about whether there are enough resources and sufficiently strong local networks to deliver public health objectives across the country (Shaw and Abbott, 2002). Public health specialists are a scarce resource. The key challenge for public health will be to be able to develop strong partnerships and alliances locally to deliver public health goals.

With the increased political focus on reducing health inequalities, the role of public health leaders has become increasingly broad and complex. Specialist public health knowledge is now just one competence that needs to be set alongside many others. These include strong management skills, the ability to work in partnership with a broad range of staff to deliver public health goals and the vision to embed public health principles into NHS organisations and a wide range of other agencies, crucially, local government.

Equally important, public health leaders must be able to work with senior NHS colleagues and local Workforce Confederation. This would ensure that the public health function (including staff such as health visitors who may not have 'public health' in their titles but who are a crucial part of the allied public health workforce) is strong enough and appropriately trained, to meet public health objectives. Finally, public health leaders need to make sure that bedrock medical public health functions, such as immunisation and screening, continue to be adequately resourced and central to public health practice.

The role of public health leaders

The key characteristic of the public health leader will be their capacity to span the medical and social dimensions of public health, to work with staff from both these perspectives to coordinate what they do. Public health leaders will be responsible for providing overviews of the health needs of their local community, paying particular attention to vulnerable groups, such as refugees and asylum seekers and travellers, or groups that have been traditionally poorly served by the NHS such as black and ethnic minority groups. Epidemiologists and information analysts will help them to collect and analyse data about local health needs and community development workers will work directly with communities so that local people's views are reflected in health needs assessments. This information will reflect not only medical need, but will also highlight areas such as environment, housing, traffic management, education and leisure services (which contribute to the 'well being' and 'quality of life'), where 'upstream interventions' could help reduce morbidity and mortality. Public health leaders will need to paint a picture of local health needs across the health economy, building strong informal health alliances and identifying local health priorities which local clinicians, health professionals and other local agencies share.

Working with PCT boards and local clinicians, they will help to assess how current services match local health need, how any identified unmet health needs will be tackled and what modifications can be made to existing services so that they reflect local need more closely. Three-year commissioning cycles will draw heavily on the quantitative and qualitative data produced through health needs assessment and public health practitioners will work closely with local acute, community and primary care providers to make sure that services respond to local need and local people's views.

Public health leaders will help set local health improvement targets which will be agreed and shared across all local agencies, including local councils, housing associations, local police forces and schools. Public health leaders will act as catalysts for action, supporting leaders and health champions in local government and beyond to understand their role in improving the health of local people. They will also monitor progress against targets and work with local media to share performance information with local people.

Staff delivering public health objectives will continue to come from a wide range of functions and perform a wide range of tasks. Public health knowledge and expertise is spread across a number of different disciplines and staff groups, including GPs, health visitors, environmental health officers, public sector researchers and community practitioners. New public health leaders will need to map out and understand this 'allied workforce', clarifying how they contribute to meeting public health goals and offering them opportunities to share existing expertise and develop new public health skills.

Public health leaders will need to create local infrastructures, or tap into existing mechanisms to communicate with, and get feedback from a broad spectrum of staff. These local structures will need to span medical interests (GPs, dentists, pharmacists, community nurses) and staff with a more social perspective (community development workers, local voluntary sector organisations and local councils). Formal structures such as PCT professional executive committees that include local GPs, nurses and professions allied to medicine and which in turn link into other professional networks may be one useful mechanism. Informal mechanisms such as lunch-time networking sessions looking a specific public health themes and targeting specific audiences may also help to bring together staff from different sectors or backgrounds who have not worked together before.

Public health leaders will need to feed intelligence gathered from these mechanisms to newly formed public health networks operating across each Strategic Health Authority area and through these, to the nine new Regional Directors of Health and Social Care.

The key skills of public health leaders

The public health leaders of the future will need to be organisational chameleons, able to operate across a wide range of settings and with a wide range of people. They will need to be comfortable operating at strategic level, making a strong case with PCT boards for local investment to meet specific health needs, identified through local needs assessment and in consultation with local communities. Equally, the new public health leader will be able to work with local voluntary sector organisations, user groups and other local community organisations to build consensus about local health priorities and to identify the best way to meet these needs. 'Walking the patch' will help them to build good relationships with local stakeholders and develop credibility with the wide range of staff (such as GPs, health visitors) that will be delivering public health objectives locally.

Public health leaders will have an important role identifying and explaining how individual staff groups contribute to public health goals. This might include working with local council housing departments to identify how they can help improve local people's health by, for example, reducing dampness, improving ventilation and fitting smoke alarms or by working with local education departments and schools to run effective sexual health programmes for young people. They will be expert influencers, able to effect change through a wide range of organisations and individuals. They will speak comfortably to others in various and different sectors (including housing construction, medicine and politics), translating public health problems and their solutions into a language all understand and feel compelled to act upon.

Joint public health appointments between primary care trusts and local authorities will become increasingly common, helping public health leaders to understand the process, functions and priorities of local government and how they can best work with these structures to implement public health goals. Relationships with local government are extremely important and public health practitioners will have a good understanding of a range of local authority functions, as well as the education sector, voluntary sector, police and fire service.

Public health leaders will need to be constantly aware of the need to identify new partners who may be able to help them develop their understanding of local health needs and to deliver public health policy locally.

As well as understanding the functions and structures of local partners, public health leaders will need to be sensitive to different organisational cultures and the different pressures and motivations in these organisations. Public health programmes will be delivered in a range of settings including GP practices, community centres, local clinics and local schools. Public health leaders will need to be able to work effectively in all these different settings and will also need to support their staff to do so as well. They will need to identify opportunities from' which public health might benefit. For example, the new health scrutiny role for local government may be one way to review a local community's health needs and other new schemes such as the New Deal for Communities programme and Neighbourhood Renewal funding, have offered new opportunities to implement health improvement objectives locally.

Public health practitioners will need strong negotiating skills. Public health will always have to compete with high-profile NHS priorities, such as reducing waiting times. Therefore, public health leaders will need to make a strong economic case for investment in health promotion and health improvement, demonstrating the potential savings to the acute sector of early intervention and prevention.

One of the most critical skills for local public health leaders will be the capacity to manage staff effectively. This will involve not only managing their own teams but also providing effective leadership and expertise to staff over whom they may have no formal managerial control. This will include staff working both in and outside the NHS. The breadth of their role will mean that they will need to be able to delegate effectively, know how to access information, experience and skills which they do not have themselves. As more public health leaders are recruited from non-medical backgrounds, it will be particularly important that they can draw on medical expertise as necessary. Public health leaders, both medical and non-medical, will need to have a sufficiently high degree of humility to accept where they need to call upon expert help and use this help appropriately.

Policy implications

Pulling together a strong public health workforce with effective local and national leaders will require consensus about the contribution that public health can make to wider public policy goals. This will require action to be taken both nationally and locally across a range of agencies.

Developing a shared set of values

Despite the increased profile of public health, there is still no consensus about the values that underpin public health as a discipline. This in part reflects the diversity of the public health workforce and the different backgrounds, professional training and values of the staff working in public health as well as the broad range of activities which fall under the umbrella of public health. It is important that a framework is developed, spelling out what drives the public health function, mapping out what it should look like and agreeing upon what criteria its successes should be judged.

Strengthening the public health workforce

Building the public health workforce of the future will need a clearer understanding of the potential contributions of a broad range of staff to meeting public health objectives. The permeability of the boundaries of public health make it difficult to assess exactly the size of the workforce but the definitions determined by the Chief Medical Officer, which identify three categories of public health implementers and influencers (see Box 1) are a useful starting point. Local public health networks will need to do more work to identify precisely which staff locally fall into which categories and to work with Workforce Confederations and local training and education bodies to fill gaps in the public health workforce.

Many PCTs are already struggling to deliver the full range of public health functions and to recruit to senior-level public health posts. Solutions such as joint health improvement posts between PCTs and local councils offer one way forward. Skills sharing between neighbouring PCTs, facilitated by public health networks is another. However, in some areas these have been slow to develop and more encouragement needs to be given to make sure that these are in place and functioning effectively.

BOX 1. The public health workforce

- a wide range of people, including managers in the NHS and local government, teachers, local business leaders and the voluntary sector who need to 'adopt a public health mindset' and to understand how their work can make a difference to local health and well-being
- a smaller number of hands-on *public health practitioners:* professionals who spend all or most of their time in public health work, including local authority environmental health officers, health visitors and those who use research or information skills working in specific public health fields
- a still smaller group of *public health specialists* working at a strategic level or senior management level or at a senior level of scientific expertise.

(Department of Health, 1998)

Improving access to training and development

PCTs will need to think creatively about how to maximise limited public health resources. Opening up public health training schemes to those without a medical background has widened the pool of people eligible for senior public health positions. However, this provides a limited number of opportunities and more needs to be done to open up access to training such as Masters in Public Health to the wider public health workforce. In addition, core public health teams should offer opportunities for staff working towards broader public health goals to work on short secondments on core public health projects to further develop their skills.

Consideration needs to be given to maximising the leadership skills of future public health leaders. Although existing masters degrees in public health and formal public health training schemes are a crucial building block for future leaders, as key components of PCT management teams, public health leaders need access to similar training opportunities such as MBA programmes or top managers schemes as to other senior NHS managers.

Building better cross-sectoral links

To meet the broad goals of public health, more work will need to go into building better links between different statutory and voluntary organisation and to develop a shared sense of local public health priorities. New Local Strategic Partnerships and the community plans that they will produce offer an excellent opportunity to develop joint health improvement goals for defined geographical areas or population groups. Shared posts such as jointly funded Directors of Public Health and health improvement are good catalysts for closer joint working. PCTs, with their local public health networks may want to consider other ways of sharing expertise and understanding between different local organisations.

Conclusion

A strong local public health function will require strong national leadership. Although the Government has undertaken a good programme of activities to reduce health inequalities, health and health improvement, one of the key planks of the public health function, remains a poor relative of health care (Appleby and Coote, 2002). The focus of Government health policy has been the NHS rather than measures to improve health. This represents a challenge for public health: should it align itself to working towards key NHS targets such as reducing avoidable cancers or should it work more widely with other local public, voluntary and private sector partners to reduce health inequalities and improve health? Refocusing public health practice equally on both these roles would require a shift in leadership by central government. This could be achieved by upgrading the role of Minister for Public Health to that of Secretary of State for Health with a junior minister retaining responsibility for the NHS. The new Secretary of State's role would include working closely with ministers in the Department for Education and Skills and Office of the Deputy Prime Minister. This would ensure that departmental policies reflect broad health improvement objectives. The Secretary of State would work with the Treasury to develop departmental health improvement targets in public service agreements, and focus policy on how to improve health, rahter than attend to the sick.

References

Acheson D (1998) *Independent Inquiry into Inequalities in Health: the Acheson Report* London: TSO

Appleby J and Coote A eds. (2002) *Five-year health check: a review of government health policy 1997-2002* London: King's Fund

Black D, Morris J, Smith C and Townsend P (1980) *Inequalities in Health: report of a research working group* London: Department of Health and Social Security

Chief Medical Officer (2001) *Getting Ahead of the Curve: a strategy for infectious diseases including other aspects of health promotion* London: Department of Health.

Department of Health (1998) *Report of Emerging Findings: Chief Medical Officer's Project to strengthen the public health function in England* London: Department of Health

Department of Health (1999) *Saving Lives: Our Healthier Nation* London: TSO

Shaw S and Abbott S (2002) Too much to handle? *Health Service Journal,* 27th June 2002 pp. 28-29

Woodhead D, Tennant R and Jochelson K (2002) *Public Health in the Balance: getting it right for London* London: King's Fund

5.The intermediate care worker

Barbara Vaughan

Executive summary

Intermediate care is based on the premise that certain patients, including those who are recuperating or who have short-term problems, may not require the facilities of an acute hospital. For these patients, recuperation could be facilitated more effectively in their homes or a similar environment.

This paper focuses on one of the key factors upon which the development of intermediate care services depends: workforce reforms. Shifting role boundaries and the development of new types of practitioners are an essential aspect of the introduction of intermediate care and are critical for effective implementation of this type of service. This paper presents a view of what shifts and roles might be required, alongside an outline of the potential barriers or obstacles to these developments. Suggestions are made for both short and long term actions required for the future.

Introduction

Background

Indications of the need for intermediate care are not hard to find. A review of surveys carried out in 20 acute hospitals in England over the past 18 months, shows an average of 29 per cent of people occupying acute hospital beds whose needs are not commensurate with that level of care (Vaughan and Withers, 2002).

Of that cohort, the reasons for ongoing admission are widespread and include 24 per cent who were awaiting long term care, 34 per cent required home or bed-based recuperation with 6 per cent requiring more complex rehabilitation. In addition there is growing concern that up to 19 per cent of those entering long term care could, within a six-month period manage more independently (Zie *et al,* 2001). This suggests that if they had been given the opportunity of access to rehabilitation then admission to a care home may, for some, have been avoided.

This picture has arisen despite the best efforts of those providing acute care. As the acuity of patients in hospital increases and the average length of stay reduces it is inevitable that priority must be given to medical crises and technical care. However, this can occur at the cost of attention to other needs such as confidence and competence building in self-care, nutritional needs and motivation. The hospital environment, with activity continuing over 24 hours, noise that will inevitably disrupt sleep, a culture of treating rather than enabling and a risk of hospital acquired infection all impede patient progress towards reaching maximum independence.

To exacerbate this problem the budget for residential and nursing home care provided through social services remains inadequate. The bed stock within nursing and residential care homes is reducing owing to an inability to continue providing services within the resources available and intensified, in mind at least, by the new regulations (Department of Health 2000). The differentiation between health and social care is vague, and there is insufficient funding to maintain mixed health and social care packages at home.

Nevertheless, despite considerable difficulties faced in implementation, pilot developments of intermediate care have been prolific throughout the UK over the past decade. Many have been highly innovative and successful at a local level (Vaughan and Lathlean 1998; Sanderson and Wright 1999), aiming to redress a situation of patient-care that is widely recognised as sub-optimal in its ability to address patients' quality of life, their choice and the financial implications of inappropriate care. Yet progress remains too slow to meet demand. Funds for intermediate care have been limited, acute care still absorbs resources, research evidence is still in its infancy and resistance to new ways of working remains high.

Models of practice for intermediate care

One of the first steps that could lead to more widespread and consistent provision of intermediate care is a realistic assessment of need. Under current classification systems, this is difficult to come by. Traditionally, patient care is packaged on the basis of clinical diagnosis. Access is provided through diagnostically grouped clinical teams and funding in acute care follows completed consultant episodes. By contrast, intermediate care services are founded on a model of health care that shifts from definition of treatment by medical diagnosis to a needs-related service. The manner in which we have traditionally 'packaged care' no longer fits. Our current classification systems do not allow for an episode of care that is related to needs, so the data that will clearly identify the extent of the problem is not available within the current coding system.

The shift that is advocated is not just an organisational change but a major alteration in culture that moves away from the traditional paradigm from which health care has been developed to a broader based model, built on a mix of health and social well being. If new services are to be developed and new roles generated accordingly, then it is critical that base level work is undertaken in both the acute sector and in the community to identify the size of the problem. Current data sets that explore delayed discharges within a narrow definition of those for whom an episode of care is completed are not sufficient. New codings are needed to encompass recuperation needs and the ability to self-care, rather than diagnosis alone.

Implications for professional education and role configuration must be considered with curriculum review to acknowledge the changing patterns of health need and reflect demographic changes in society (see below).

Professional roles

At present

There is no doubt that the current inter and intra-professional divisions of labour inhibit the successful move to intermediate care. Health practitioner roles have developed within tightened boundaries defining what it is legitimate for nurses, GPs, therapists, and others to do. This distinction of roles has most frequently been differentiated by the development of a false care (nurses, therapists) and cure (GPs, physicians, surgeons) divide. This situation is exacerbated by the proliferation of new groups, both within each occupational structure and independently, all of which has led to a highly specialist but often reductionist approach to care. Over time the subdivisions in each of these groups has become exacerbated by the prolific increase in knowledge, which has, in turn impacted on structures and services.

While the value of specialist care should never be underestimated nothing comes without a price. Within intermediate care the difficulties caused by division of labour are, at one level, simplistic, but at another they can put very real barriers in the way of progress. At the simplest level, access to equipment can be hampered by the traditional interpretation of role boundaries while at a more critical level the authority to manage care can be delayed through lack of authority and autonomy for some team members. For example authority to admit and discharge from a service has traditionally been vested in medicine (Read *et al,* 1999), while in intermediate care this may be more appropriately managed through a hybrid of therapists and nurses.

It should be stressed that the division of labour, including gate keeping to services, has developed through time and practice rather than any more logical reason but is deemed by many practitioners and managers to be unalterable. At one end are concerns about territory and control, at the other are fears of error.

To a large extent the workforce has become disabled by its own presumptions, with general practitioners concerned that they alone will take the work burden of intermediate care. Nurses and therapists are concerned about the new areas of responsibility and accountability, such as the loss of the blanket of false protection from medicine. Social workers may be preoccupied with a presumption that they and they alone are concerned about social well-being (Vaughan and Steiner, 1999).

The critical factor for intermediate care is that the group of patients served require skills which are currently shared between different disciplines and supplied though different agencies. For example: whilst it is an occupational therapist who may be responsible for assessing home adaptation for a patient which will then be supplied through local authority agencies, help with mobility may be vested with physiotherapists. While it is the nursing team who help with dressings and hygiene, it is social service carers who provide meals and home care. The transition of medical care between hospital and community doctors occurs at a different point in the clinical pathway and some have suggested that this is outside the usual General Medical Services remit. Requests for readmission may come from a non-medical member of the intermediate care team, breaking the customary referral pathway. Hence the current division of labour between the different occupational groups is no longer workable.

The implications for shared working and the development of 'roles fit for purpose' are self-evident. It is no longer viable or acceptable for each occupational group within the traditional team to retain control over the aspects of work that have, often through time and practice rather than logic or knowledge, become the province of that group. We have neither the workforce nor the resources to maintain that approach to service delivery. More importantly, duplication of effort on the part of the professional care-givers is well recognised by patients who are themselves partners in this process.

They can, and do, become frustrated by delay caused by need for referral through another route; by the need to retell the same story; by conflicting messages, and by lack of continuity. Thus if there is to be real change in practice, then a fundamental pre-requisite is to review the team roles and structures, alongside authority and responsibility for practice, and areas of autonomy and accountability.

What is required?

In developing teams for intermediate care it is critical to differentiate between *multi*-professional and *inter*-professional working, recently raised by the Department of Health (Department of Health, 2000). Multi-professional working brings together a group that works collaboratively but within which members retain their separate divisions of labour, knowledge and professional identity. With inter-professional working there is a willingness to share expertise and knowledge across traditional boundaries in order to meet needs within a particular service framework more effectively (Masterson, 2002).

For intermediate care multi-professional working is not an option - since it does not provide for patient-centred need but retains a service driven by professional structures and boundaries. Recognition of this change at a strategic level is slow to emerge, with unions and the Royal Colleges lagging behind in their response to this area of clinical need. Similarly, in education the activity has largely taken place at a repair level with post-graduate courses to prepare people fit for a role, but with little attention paid as yet to entry to the professions, possibly because this is just too hard. Thus despite the best efforts many fundamental principles related to current practice remain un-addressed.

What might an effective intermediate carer role look like?

At an operational level, however, there are some excellent examples of effective inter-professional practice where obstacles have been overcome. The essence of these developments has been that roles have developed around patient need, unhampered by boundary concerns but focusing on the ability to provide continuity of care and reduce overlap of effort and delay.

The aim of role development is that within an intermediate care team, any qualified team member can undertake an overview assessment, taking into account the range of skills which each occupational group can offer, as well as the priorities of the patient. The critical factor is to be able to identify what is within the range of 'usual care' and the point at which a referral may be required for a specific occupational group for specialist assessment (Department of Health, 2000). For example, a nurse, therapist or general practitioner can undertake a basic assessment of mobility (one of the most frequently seen needs in intermediate care settings) and set in place a programme of care. In turn, this may be implemented in conjunction with the patient, carer and generic care assistant. However should the difficulty with mobility be more complex referral may be needed to the GP for medicines review or the physiotherapist for work with balance.

To achieve this end (from the current starting point of separate occupational groups with their own requirements for entry to the profession) both knowledge and the development of skills must be shared between team members. For example the occupational therapists may share knowledge of the range of simple home adaptations and the way in which they can be accessed. The GP may help other team members learn simple chest percussion skills in order that they can monitor home care effectively. As pathways of care are developed and the confidence and competence of the team grows, deficits in knowledge of the groups concerned will become apparent, which can then be corrected by either in house or modular training programmes based on clinical need rather than professional boundaries.

Steps towards operationalising professional roles

There are several steps that could be taken by Government, Workforce Development Confederations and Trusts to aid the development of intermediate care roles without the necessity of reviewing entry to professional groups. In the first instance the Government should provide clarification both professionally and legally for any areas of care which must be confined to a particular occupational group. In practice there are very few tasks that are limited to occupational groups since the essence of professional practice should be based on knowledge and judgement, neither of which can be monopolised by a single group. However local insight and variations are widespread and wider guidance would be of value.

Following from this, wider debate about the development of shared occupational standards is needed in order to begin to break down the lack of understanding between the different professional groups and identify opportunities for shared learning at undergraduate rather than post graduate level. Fear that this could lead to an emphasis on training for tasks rather than the development of problem-solving skills would need to be confronted.

Flexible post-graduate courses that allow for the development of knowledge and skills related to role are also urgently needed. These would have a common route of entry and the opportunity to challenge for mastery, which may have been achieved through experience. A further feature of post-graduate training must be the facility for practitioners to shift horizontally between different occupational groups to allow for skills-development according to role. This would, ideally, replace the need to re enter a new training programme at the base level, allowing for cost saving by building on current knowledge rather than presuming that all subject areas must be re-addressed.

Finally, however, a review of entry to professional groups and current division of labour is critical.

The wider implications of new roles

Workforce Planning

Throughout health and social care there are concerns about recruitment and retention. Staff shortages are closely linked to weaknesses in workforce planning arrangements: the mechanism that is intended to ensure that adequate numbers or practitioners, with the appropriate skills, are available to deliver patient care. It is clear that an approach to workforce planning that begins by assessing the shortfall in known current roles such as hospital doctors, general practitioners, or nurses will not lead to the emergence and training of intermediate care workers. If we are to overcome the challenges we know must be addressed in both acute and primary care then workforce planning systems must take account of new roles and related clinical career pathways. To this end, structural divisions in workforce planning which separate medicine from other occupational groups must be addressed.

It would aid workforce planning further if research was conducted to establish whether recruitment and retention levels in intermediate care teams are higher than average. Within many of the early intermediate pilot sites recruitment was not a problem as the sites gained the reputation of being 'a good place to work' (personal communication). However, there is an argument that pilot schemes are usually run by well-motivated enthusiastic teams who are fun to work with. There is also a case for suggesting that there was a more fundamental cultural change occurring in these units. While we prepare most health and social care practitioners to degree level or beyond, we do not create the roles that allow them to exercise clinical judgement that is commensurate with their levels of knowledge and competency. Nor do we allow them the autonomy to carry a patient case-load and manage some aspects of care independently. Thus the situation has arisen where one arm of the workforce (GPs) is at risk of role overload while another (nurses and therapists), despite potentially having appropriate knowledge and skills, is denied the freedom to practice and is at risk of both boredom and frustration within the work place.

For some, working in intermediate care can help to overcome these problems. The softening of role boundaries has allowed for more fulfilling work, unhampered by delays to practice. Through skill sharing better continuity is obtained with greater job satisfaction.

Fears of missed pathology

One danger that is often highlighted in discussions about possible increases in domiciliary care, or bed-based care in non-acute settings as advocated by enthusiasts for intermediate care, is the risk of missing underlying pathology (Bulger, 2002). Concerns are frequently directed towards the capabilities of non-medical members of the team in relation to managing care for people with undifferentiated diagnosis. However, it is usually these team members who alert medical colleagues for the need for action or investigation, requesting expert advice and sometimes initiating investigation (Evans and Griffiths 1994).

Whilst there are arguments for and against the development of guidelines and the more prescriptive protocols, these can offer a safeguard if used in conjunction with single assessment processes and learning opportunities. The critical issue here is to ensure dedicated time for learning in order that guidelines are a tool rather than a master and can direct people to appropriate pathways according to need, including access to expert advice.

It is also important that referral must be available to all members of an *inter*disciplinary intermediate care team to same day or rapid access *multi* disciplinary clinics where the 'expert' aspects of the different roles can be accessed speedily under one roof. To this end new knowledge related to diagnostics and referral pathways may need to be developed by some team members.

Litigation

It has been the tradition of professions to be judged through peer review by members of their own profession in questions of professional error and by law if actions may have been criminal. With the emergence of hybrid roles, serious questions, as yet unanswered, arise about the standards by which practitioners will be judged. The classic guidance in medicine has been to judge by Bolam standards, that is judged by a peer group from the same discipline, but acceptability of this approach as new roles are developing must be challenged.

The first step towards minimisation of patient-risk is continual professional development for all practitioners. Yet this has to be relevant. It is inadequate to attend accredited learning sessions unless the relevance to practice can be clearly identified and linked to necessary change in behaviour. The advent of appraisal in general practice only touches the tip of this iceberg in terms of the need for assessment and skills development and there is a strong case for much tighter regulation of learning for all team members.

As inter-disciplinary teams develop appraisal, clinical supervision and individual performance review should be pre-requisites, linked to performance targets. To help these emerging teams, clear guidance about the ways in which cases should be handled, developed by multi-professional groups, is urgently required.

Employment contracts

As interagency and inter-disciplinary working develops, the anomalies that lie between groups and employers become evident. Terms and conditions of employment may vary, as can requirements for the maintenance of professional competence. Ways have been found at a local level for overcoming at least some of these problems by, for example, sharing or pooling of budgets and using one agency through which all employment is managed. However agreements are time consuming to manage, with concerns on all sides about, for example, professional identity, cost implications, protection of the public and of the staff.

In order for intermediate care to progress at the local level, lack of equity between public agencies in relation to personnel policies must be addressed and common ground needs to be found. Terms of employment should be uniform for all employing agencies.

Conculsion

Intermediate care offers real hope for the future, providing a service that is sensitive to need, at or near home, goal directed and aimed at maximising independence and the ability to self-care. Early studies suggest that outcomes from such services are as good or better than acute care management with an added factor of high patient satisfaction (Wilson *et al,* 1999; Richards *et al,* 1998). The driving forces behind this initiative are to provide care specific to the needs of a medically stable or predictable group of patients who have the potential to regain a greater degree of independence. The starting point is not the issue of reducing so called 'bed blocking'. Though currently this may be a motivator high on the minds of some, programmes are doomed to fail if the original intention behind the service development becomes lost in managerial and organisational targets.

Within this framework an exploration of role function is essential to success. The current divisions of labour within and between occupational groups and agencies are major barriers to successful implementation. While many teams have found short-term solutions, working collaboratively, sharing budgets, sharing skills and working to a common purpose, the underlying issues of interdisciplinary working remain problematic.

If the cultural change that underpins intermediate care is to be effectively addressed then implications for professional education, assurance of competence, clinical career paths, employment conditions and authority and autonomy for practice must be acknowledged and addressed at local and national levels.

References

Bulger G (2002) 'Intermediate Care is Ageist' *British Medical Journal* 8th June 2002.

Department of Health (2000) *A health service for all talents: report on the review of workforce planning* London: TSO

Department of Health (2000) *Care Homes for Older People National Minimum Standards* London: Department of Health [www.doh.gov.uk/ncsc]

Department of Health (2001) Health Services/Local Authority Circular HSC 2001/1 *Intermediate Care* 19th January 01, London: Department of Health

Department of Health (2000) *National Service Framework for Older People* London: TSO

Evans A and Griffiths P (1994) *The Development of a Nursing-Led In-Patient Service* London King's Fund

Masterson A (2002) 'Cross boundary working: a macro-political analysis of the impact on professional roles' *Journal of Clinical Nursing* 11(3) pp 331- 339

Read S, Doyal L and Vaughan B (1999) *Exploring new roles in practice: implications of developments within the clinical team (ENRiP)* Sheffield: School of Health & Related Research (ScHARR), University of Sheffield

Richards S *et al* (1998) 'Randomised controlled trial comparing effectiveness and acceptability of an early discharge, hospital at home scheme with acute hospital care' *British Medical Journal* 1998: 316 pp1796-1801

Sanderson D and Wright D (1999) *Final evaluation of the CARATS initiatives in Rotheram* York: University of York Health Economics Consortium

Vaughan B and Lathlean J (1998) *Intermediate Care : models in practice,* London: Kings Fund

Vaughan B and Withers G (2002) 'Acute Distress' *Health Service Journal* 112 (5804) May 9, 2002 pp 24-27

Vaughan B and Steiner A (1999) *The shape of the team* London: Kings Fund

Wilson, A *et al* (1999) 'Randomised controlled trial of effectiveness of Leicester hospital at home scheme compared with hospital care' *British Medical Journal* 1999:319 pp1542-1546

Zie H *et al* (2001) 'Modeling decisions of a multi disciplinary panel for admission to long term care' *Health Care Management Science* Vol. 4 issue 4

6. The lay person as healthcare practitioner

by Stephen Fishwick and Melinda Letts

Executive summary

The NHS Plan refers throughout to the need to develop a genuinely patient centred service (Department of Health, 2000). This will require some painful reflection about whether NHS resources are spent on the things that make the most difference to patients and their quality of life. It will mean careful consideration of how patients are involved in decisions about their own treatment, together with funding for information provision and support for self-care.

This paper aims to stimulate thinking about the role that people with long term conditions play as 'patient practitioners'. It sets out the current extent of patients' participation in health care and explores some of the policy changes that might facilitate an increased role while guarding against the risks involved.

Introduction

Being a patient is not a permanent status. Many people who have been acutely ill but recover are patients for only a brief period. Likewise, many of those suffering from a long-term medical condition do not think of themselves as 'patients' except on the occasions they are actually in hospital or consulting a health professional. Yet the NHS has long been organised around people's needs only at these points in time. This is beginning to change. The NHS Plan aspires to a future in which 'the NHS becomes a resource that people routinely use every day to help them look after themselves' (Department of Health, 2000). It must become a service that helps people to maintain their own health, staffed by healthcare practitioners skilled at supporting people in the management of their own conditions.

This calls for a new style of interaction between professionals and people using the NHS. Efficient partnerships will involve professionals overseeing as much as, if not more than, administering care. The aim is not that patients usurp the professional's role but that patients should be seen as, in some respects, practitioners in their own right. Achieving this will necessitate real commitment to developing people's own skills in self-care and to changing the way in which they are seen and treated by health professionals.

People with long-term conditions are particularly well placed to benefit from this approach. This paper aims to stimulate thinking about the role that people with long-term conditions play as patients or lay practitioners. It sets out the current extent of patients' participation in health care and explores some of the policy changes that might facilitate an increased role while guarding against the risks involved.

What is meant by self-management?

Self-management and self-care can take numerous different forms (the terms here are used interchangeably for simplicity's sake). The narrowest definition refers to structured self-management programmes.[1] However, using the broadest interpretation, self-care constitutes around 90 per cent of all health care (Department of Health, 2002). This figure incorporates practices such as self-monitoring for emergency care (it is estimated that more than one million people in the UK currently use a community alarm system at home) and the management of long-term conditions.

Self-management for a person with diabetes may involve the person adhering to an appropriate diet, monitoring glucose levels and self-administering insulin. Someone with asthma may be involved in self-management through aiming to understand and avoid things that trigger their asthma, monitoring their peak flow and, within the framework of a care plan agreed with their heath professional, taking preventive medication as necessary.

Lay-led self-management operates on the basis that a person with personal experience of a chronic condition may be well placed to help others, due to the expertise gained through living with a day-to-day routine of self-management. A current example is Project Dil, operating within the Leicester Health Action Zone, which aims to prevent coronary heart disease and diabetes. Voluntary peer educators, trained to educate about diet and exercise, each deliver 45 hours of health education activities including healthy cookery demonstrations, walking groups, smoking cessation talks, and visits to temples and mosques to provide information about heart disease.

Benefits of self-care

Health and lifestyle

People with long-term conditions have long recognised that the day-to-day management of their condition is a key determinant of their quality of life. It is clear that self-care can improve the quality of this day-to-day management.

The Chronic Disease Self-Management Course (CDSMC), evaluated within the Living with Long-term Illness (LILL) project was shown to lead to a range of improvements for patients. These included: an increase in self-efficacy (perception of disease control); improved cognitive symptom management (use of self-management techniques); improved communication with physician, reduced health distress and fatigue; improvement in anxious mood; improved symptom control and shortness of breath, and improved mental health. Training in self-management programmes at early stages of a condition may also help prevent the onset of multiple complications and further disability in later life (Department of Health, 2002).

The benefits are not confined to patient education programmes. Millions of people daily make informed choices about their lifestyle and their care, thereby taking various degrees of control over their condition. Where people with diabetes take on greater responsibility for the management of their condition, they have shown health outcome benefits in terms of reduced blood glucose levels, with no increase in severe hypoglycaemic attacks. They have also indicated a marked improvement in quality of life and a significant increase in satisfaction with treatment (Department of Health, 2001a). Self-management amongst asthma outpatients has been shown to reduce symptoms, emergency visits to GPs, hospitalisation and days off work (Gibson *et al,* 1999). The experience is similarly positive in numerous other disease groups.

Workforce pressures

With an ageing population presenting a growing challenge to NHS human resource capacity, it makes sense to add people with personal experience of long term conditions to the skill-mix in primary care. The Wanless report considered staffing and skill substitution until 2020. It suggested that nurse practitioners could undertake 20 per cent of the work of doctors which would help solve the doctor shortage but create a nursing gap that could be only partially compensated for by accelerated recruitment of healthcare assistants (Wanless, 2002). Commentators argue that, 'this pinpoints the HR crunch factor - to change the NHS workforce, we also need to grow it' (Buchan, 2002). People with long-term conditions undoubtedly provide a rich source of untapped capacity for the health service. They are numerous, highly motivated, expert in what it means to live with a chronic condition and, relative to salaried staff, carry little cost.

The potential for patients to relieve a hard-pressed NHS workforce should not, however, be exaggerated. To be effective and safe, self-care requires a considerable commitment from the health professional. Guided self-management increases the call on health professionals' time at the start of the treatment process in particular.

Cost-effective care

The quid pro quo is that self-management may lead to more informed and appropriate use of health and social care services as people feel more in control of their condition (Department of Health, 2002). Where patients' ownership of decision making about their course of treatment increases, so does medical concordance, resulting in better clinical outcomes. The Royal Pharmaceutical Society of Great Britain identified how concordance might reduce preventable illness and avoidable hospital admissions and wasted medicines (Royal Pharmaceutical Society of Great Britain, 1997).

Greater openness and trust between patients and health professionals might have still wider advantages. Honest discussion about risk, responsibility and rationing could extrapolate into more realistic understanding and expectations about what the health service can deliver. In short, 'grown up' relationships between patients and health professionals should result in a more mature relationship between the public and the health service.

The Hypothetical Journey of an 'Expert Patient'

Leanne Jones [30] has lived with arthritis for the past 10 years and with asthma since childhood. Five years ago Leanne was almost housebound, her confidence had been eroded to the point where she felt unable to be away from home for more than a few hours. A friend told Leanne about a self-management course she had attended, run by a local charity. The course was about helping people manage their lives with long-term conditions whatever these were. Leanne went along. She found that the course helped her to be more confident when talking with her GP, her consultants and asthma nurse about the problems she was having. In effect, the course had provided her with a toolkit of techniques for her to use on a daily basis to help her feel more in control of the ups and downs of living with her long-term conditions. Most importantly Leanne felt that she wasn't alone.

Five years on, Leanne still uses many of the techniques taught on the course such as goal setting, positive self-talk and distraction to help her when things get bad. She is busier and experiences less fatigue and pain. She has a pretty good idea of her plans for the year and now works part-time. The techniques work well to help her manage her arthritis pain so she does not need to take as many painkillers. This is also good for her asthma.

Her GP has also seen the difference, and feels confident in Leanne's ability to know what is best for her. She is happy to work in partnership with Leanne to support the medical management of her arthritis and monitor her asthma plan. Leanne has not had a 'flare up' for a good few years, but still meets with her rheumatologist once a year and knows that she can contact him directly by phone or email if she needs to. She also makes use of the advice of her local pharmacist when she is unsure about some of her medication. Initially she had to tell him about self-management courses, but now he knows all about them. He includes details of local courses when dispensing drugs to his other clients living with long-term illnesses.

The personal organiser Leanne was given a few years ago enables her to keep a record of her medication usage and her 'ups and downs'. Leanne has become good friends with two people from the course and they still encourage and support each other. She has also spoken at local meetings organised by the NHS Expert Patients Programme to tell others what a turning point the course was in her life. After one of these meetings she was asked if she would like to join her local Patients Forum.

Necessary changes in policy and practice

In July 1999 the Government published its White Paper *Saving Lives: Our Healthier Nation* (Department of Health, 1999). The paper explained that one of the Government's intentions was to help people living with long term illness maintain their health and improve their quality of life through an Expert Patients Programme. A Task Force was set up to design such a programme.

The Expert Patients Programme

The Department of Health-sponsored Expert Patients Programme attempts to develop a health service support mechanism for self-management of chronic conditions or disabilities, including asthma, diabetes, MS, sickle cell disease, hearing and sight impairments. The Expert Patients Taskforce noted that, although people have educational needs specific to their individual disease, they also have common requirements, for example:

- knowing how to recognise and act upon symptoms
- dealing with acute attacks or exacerbations of the disease
- making the most effective use of medicines and treatment
- understanding the implications of professional advice
- establishing a stable pattern of sleep and rest and dealing with fatigue
- accessing social services
- managing work and the resources of employment services
- accessing chosen leisure activities
- developing strategies to deal with the psychological consequences of illness learning to cope with other people's response to their chronic illness

(Department of Health, 2001b).

Such initiatives are necessary, however they are not sufficient to achieve a step-change in the level of self-care activity. They remain small scale (the budget for the Expert Patients Programme is only £3million) and are just one part of the more far-reaching and fundamental re-negotiation of the relationship between patient and professional that is now required.

Changing culture

The still dominant stereotype of the health professional is of someone who talks about rather than with the patient and to whom patients are interesting mainly as embodiments of their conditions. Health professionals are under immense pressure and have little time to engage in dialogue with patients. Meanwhile, there remains something of a culture of deference to medical authority and many patients still do not see a role for themselves beyond 'doing what they're told'. This may be particularly true for older patients who tend to regard moves towards giving patients greater responsibility for their health as about cutting corners and saving money rather than improving patient care (Edwards 2001). Clearly, all of this inhibits self-care. Health professionals must increasingly share knowledge with the patient, discuss options for care and even cede responsibility for making key health decisions. In return, patients (indeed all of us) must understand that our responsibilities to ourselves, our children or whoever else on whose behalf we are seeking advice cannot be left at the surgery door.

Under this model, health professionals can be viewed as professional advisers in (probably most of) our interactions with them, resembling other professionals from whom we take advice. We go to a solicitor, for example, to take advantage of the professional knowledge they have amassed. We expect them to keep up to date through continuing professional education. But the decisions we make following a consultation are our responsibility, not theirs. If they advise us badly and we can prove that they should have known better, then we can complain, and if they have given us advice that has a catastrophic effect they may be penalised for negligence.

In this new type of relationship, health professionals cannot be blamed if patients in the full knowledge of the implications refuse specific treatments. Patient choices may be clinically sub-optimal. For example, in diabetes people may choose to run their blood sugars slightly high because they are more worried about the short-term impact of hypoglycaemia on their day-to-day quality of life than they are about long term complications. Nor can health professionals be expected to know everything all the time. It has to be made acceptable for them to say 'I don't know'. They may then also be more likely to work with the patient to determine the relevant facts and/or solutions.

If health professionals are willingly to share ownership of care but remain appropriately accountable for the part they play in decisions that are made, the NHS must be protected from the excesses of the blame and litigation culture reaching these shores from across the Atlantic. Currently, 28,000 people make written complaints about aspects of their treatment in hospitals each year and the bill for negligence claims is some £400 million. Medical negligence rules might usefully be reformed to incorporate the concept of 'mediation', which is discussed below.

Mediation

Mediation is a process used for resolving disputes outside the traditional legal system where the services of an independent and specially trained third party (the mediator) are employed to facilitate the negotiation and resolution of the dispute. Benefits of mediation are that it substantially reduces the dispute cycle time and costs of resolution and more importantly that the parties maintain responsibility and control for the outcome which may involve the examination and consideration of wider needs and interests rather than focussing purely on financial compensation.

Mediation has an 85 per cent success rate and a high post dispute satisfaction rate – in that it establishes a learning as opposed to an adversarial environment. Rather than being placed in a position that requires them to defend behaviour and attitudes, both practitioner and patient frequently value the opportunity to establish dialogue in a safe and structured forum that enables them to explore why the dispute arose in the first place.

(Gunn, 2002).

Policy recommendations

Only when the concept of shared ownership is comfortable for and accepted by the whole health community – health professionals, patients and managers – can the various practical steps towards enabling self-care achieve their full potential.

Educating professionals

Professional training will, in future, need to place greater emphasis on supporting self-care, particularly for people with long-term conditions. The proposals already being developed as a result of the NHS Plan do not go far enough. Professional education needs genuinely to reflect the new commitment to a patient centred health service, with professionals being taught to value patients' views and to understand the contribution patients can make to 'best care'. While health professionals provide general information about conditions and their symptoms and can generalise about the benefits and side effects of different treatment options, patients (if allowed and encouraged) can explain the effects of the condition on their life and the impact of different treatment options on their enjoyment of life.

Preparing patients

Patients may be anxious about carrying more responsibility for health and managing uncertainty, and they also need to be reassured. The improved health outcomes seen among motivated patients in evaluated courses such as CDSMC will translate into the general population only if patients are made aware of the benefits and, importantly, convinced about their own validity as decision makers. Reliable information upon which to make decisions is a crucial element of the process. Health professionals are still by far the most trusted source of health information (Edwards, 2001), sometimes to the exclusion of other sources. This is why the question of validation must be addressed, whether the sources are NHS service providers, commercial outlets, the World Wide Web or community pharmacists (Department of Health, 2002).

Incentivising managers

Meanwhile, NHS managers need to be permitted to shift their focus from patching people up in acute care. Performance targets and resources emanating from the centre still fail to reward attempts to secure a higher quality of life for people who can't be cured. Current systems of evaluation, firmly focused on activity rates in secondary care, present a partial and not necessarily helpful picture. For example, it may be valuable to know how efficient hospital care is, but for a measure of how effective our health care system is we need to know how many people could have been prevented from needing hospital care in the first place. Measurements related to increased levels of patient involvement and quality of life outcomes should receive higher recognition. The National Director for Mental Health recently acknowledged the validity of subjective measures of success by calling for data covering quality of life and users/carers' satisfaction to sit alongside data for mortality and morbidity.[2]

Some Steps Towards Patients as Lay Practitioners

- Jointly agreed personal care plans should become the norm. These are negotiated and agreed following a full discussion of the choices between the patient and the healthcare professional involved in their care. The care plan should then be included in a patient held record.
- Self-management courses. These can be made much more widely available, and it is vital that the voluntary sector remains involved and consulted so that the roll-out of self-management does not become divorced from the cumulative expertise developed in the sector over a decade or so. Many patient groups are, however, under-resourced and groups do not exist for all conditions. Thereafter, sustained investment in patient education that is structured, ongoing, consistent, up-to-date and person-centred will need to be a permanent feature of primary care provision.
- Emphasis on patient-friendly forums, such as community pharmacy. Pharmacists have a key role to play in self-care, for example in managing repeat prescribing aided by electronic heath records (Department of Health, 2000).
- Better access to health information through, for example, an expansion of NHS Direct. The IPPR, for one, has suggested a ring-fenced budget to ensure high quality, timely information to become available to patients: 'Improving information for patients must be seen as a core health service issue, not an optional extra' (Kendall, 2001).
- Investment in portable/remote diagnostic and treatment equipment. This may allow patients' homes to become the key site of healthcare delivery within 15 years (Robert, 1999).

Conclusion

A shift towards greater patient involvement has already begun and the trend is likely to continue, as much due to demographic and cultural processes as to policies directed from above (Department of Health, 2001b). Take an affluent, consumer society with a lot of information and the means to broadcast it easily. Add an unprecedented amount of interest in individual health and opportunities to spend money on it. Result: a much more demanding, more discriminating body of NHS users. The current older generation, with their innate sense that the NHS is something to be grateful for and their received belief that doctor knows best, are no longer the people who shape how Britain perceives its health service. The future elderly may be better equipped and more inclined to join the skills mix. This generation's consumerist tendencies can be a driver for positive change, but must be channelled towards constructive, efficient patient-professional partnerships.

References

Department of Health (1999), *Saving Lives: Our Healthier Nation* London: TSO

Department of Health (2000) *The NHS Plan: A Plan for Investment. A Plan for Reform* London: TSO

Department of Health (2001a) *National Service Framework for Diabetes: Standards* London: TSO

Department of Health (2001b) *The Expert Patient: A New Approach to Chronic Disease Management for the 21st Century,* London: TSO

Department of Health (2002) *Strategies to Support Self-care: Next Steps workshop background paper* London: Department of Health (unpublished)

Edwards L (2001) *The Future of Healthcare: the Patient Perspective in England*: London: Institute for Public Policy Research (unpublished) http://www.ippr.org.uk/research/index.php?current=22&project=48

Gunn J. (2002) *Alternative Dispute Resolution (ADR) in a value chain transformed by on-line transactions NHS Mediator* London: January 2002 (www.corpeace.com).

Kendall L. (2001) *The Future Patient* London: Institute for Public Policy Research

Robert G. (1999) *Science & Technology; trends and issues forward to 2015: implications for healthcare* Policy Future for UK Health Technical Series, London: Nuffield Trust

Royal Pharmaceutical Society of Great Britain (1997) *From Compliance to Concordance: Achieving Shared Goals in Decision Taking* London: Royal Pharmaceutical Society of Great Britain

Wanless (2002) *Securing Our Future Health: Taking a Long Term View* London: TSO

Wyatt, J C (1998) 'Four Barriers to Realising the Information Revolution in Health Care', in Lenaghan J (ed) (1998) *Rethinking IT and Health* London: Institute for Public Policy Research

Williams S, Weinman J and Dale J (1998) 'Doctor patient communication and patient satisfaction: a review' *Family Practice* 8: 237-242

Acknowledgements: with thanks to Jane Cooper, Long Term Medical Conditions Alliance for her contribution of the 'Hypothetical Journey of an Expert Patient' case study.

1 Self management programmes: In the UK, from the mid-1990s onwards, organisations supporting people with long term conditions, such as Arthritis Care and the Manic Depression Fellowship increasingly embraced the concept of lay led self management as a means to enable people with long term conditions to take greater control over their own lives. It was in this context that the Long-term Medical Conditions Alliance began the Living with Long-term Illness (LILL) project in September 1998. Its remit was to increase the availability of lay led self-management for people with long term conditions and build effective partnerships between patients, voluntary organisations and health professionals.

2 Established tools include the Manchester Short Assessment of Quality of Life (Mansa) and the Carers and Users Expectation of Services (Cues).

7. Knowledge brokers as change agents

Dr Cecilia Pyper

Executive summary

This paper suggests that, as internet access and IT technology develop, the challenge for both patients and professionals will be accessing relevant health information and exchanging and communicating that information in a way that meets patients needs and promotes the most efficient use of services. As one way of meeting these challenges, it proposes the exploration of 'knowledge brokers' – practitioners who work with particular patient groups or communities to promote dissemination of knowledge, to support healthy life-style practices, the self-management of certain minor and chronic conditions, improved understanding about the management of chronic conditions and how to access local services appropriately.

Introduction

> Give a person a fish, and you feed him for a day. Teach a person to fish, you feed them for a lifetime. (Chinese proverb)

Knowledge is the currency of the new millennium. The challenge now faced by NHS professionals and patients is not an information shortage but information overload. The new workforce capacity required within the NHS and social services is in practitioners who are able to identify and respond to different user groups' information needs and who have the skill to identify and to refine this information.

In order for information and communication technologies to become empowerment tools, global information must be matched by access to relevant national and local information in a format that patients find useful. It is highly significant that one of the suggested reasons that there is little evidence of the effects of Internet information on health outcomes (Bessell *et al,* 2002) is that there are insufficient mechanisms for identifying quality sources of information (Risk *et al,* 2001).

So one challenge for the future is to ensure that information is local and relevant for patients. Primary care centres, hospitals, and healthcare trusts are independent organisations with independent information systems. This frequently results in patients having difficulty accessing clear information when they are receiving an integrated care package from more than one organisation or are being transferred from hospital to the home care services. It is essential that there is a local strategy for co-ordinating this information and ensuring it is consistent and regularly updated.

It is also important to recognise that social inequalities have given rise to the 'digital divide,' that prevent certain groups of society having access to these new knowledge banks (Parent *et al,* 2001).

Action is needed to ensure that ensure that practitioners can help to bridge this divide. This does not necessarily mean extra work for existing NHS and social care staff. Many health professionals are not trained to address the wider areas that influence people's health, including their emotional and social wellbeing. Although some health problems certainly require sophisticated health management from highly trained heath professionals, others can be more appropriately managed at lower cost outside the traditional management structures of the NHS.

The Wanless Report, commissioned by the Treasury, is the first ever evidence-based assessment of the long-term resource requirements for the NHS. It draws attention to the potential significance of self-care in this respect (a theme further developed by Barbara Vaughn in Chapter 5 of this publication). Encouraging citizens to become accustomed to practising health seeking behaviour and self-care has become fundamental to ensuring in the future that effective services can be delivered by the NHS.

In summary there are three stages required for the NHS to improve knowledge management:

- knowledge production: producing the knowledge required by commissioning relevant research, development and evaluation;
- knowledge appraisal: determining the quality and relevance of information;
- knowledge distribution: ensuring new knowledge is made available in a useful format to the relevant user professional or patient groups.

The key challenges that face the NHS and must be met in order for the benefits of the increasing knowledge base to be realised by the patients/citizens are:

- ensuring that patients/citizens have access to relevant national and local information;
- ensuring that patients/citizens have equality of access to quality information sources;
- providing information sources that integrate and cater for the breath of patients/citizens different needs;
- enabling patients/citizens to participate safely and actively in shared management or self-care.

The challenge now for the NHS is to establish the mind-set and workforce that can bring about the necessary changes in attitudes and service delivery. Central to this is the development of new skills within the NHS and social services workforce as well as the introduction of additional skills from outside the workforce in order to create expertise in 'knowledge brokering'. This paper considers the range of 'knowledge brokers', formed both from within and outside the medical community, who could help the NHS to meet the challenges outlined above.[2]

The role(s) of knowledge brokers

Some knowledge brokers will require specialised skills training, such as IT/counselling or will perform more effectively if they are closely linked to specific services. Other practitioners need to be more eclectic and responsive to their clients needs, using a variety of facilitation skills. Some will be employed within primary care practices or across PCTs and Local Authorities, others may work within voluntary or disease-specific organisations. To illustrate these different roles a series of case scenarios will describe the range of knowledge brokers required in order to allow for the evolution of more informed and independent patients.

Peer knowledge brokers

Peer knowledge brokers are individuals who are close in background or age to groups that have a specific requirement and may be excluded from access to general information. Peer knowledge brokers gain additional skills that equip them to work in partnership with their clients and enable/ facilitate the process of translating reliable information into a form that their clients find useful. They may be appointed to co-ordinate an existing group of patients or service users – or may actively draw together a real or virtual group of people with similar circumstances, such as young care leavers or mothers suffering from post-natal depression. Through working with service users to locate, filter and disseminate helpful information the peer knowledge broker has the potential to build skills within their clients groups so that in many situations some responsibility for managing new information devolves to the group with the ongoing support or supervision of the knowledge broker.

One example of peer knowledge brokers working in practice is a current teenage and young parents networking website project that has been developed by the users/parents themselves with the support of facilitators in Oxford and Great Yarmouth. The facilitators have been local and of a similar age to the young parents. They have worked with individuals, groups and health professionals to develop a website that is relevant to needs of teenage parents in general and to the specific health, social and educational services offered in their local area. The lessons learnt, so far, are that the process of developing modifying and updating the website has been as important to the clients as the information itself. The subject matter conveyed on the website has initiated further discussions and exploration of issues of concern to the clients. In this example additional facilities are now being developed to enable transfer some of the of IT skills to the clients so that this specific group can continue to build or amend the website.[3]

IT knowledge brokers

IT knowledge brokers work with patients and either access information on their behalf or teach patients how to use computers and access websites and use simple search methodologies. These knowledge brokers require good interpersonal skills and computer skills. They will have an ever-increasing role in the NHS enabling patients who are unfamiliar with computers or the Internet to access health information of access their electronic health record.

The emergence of IT knowledge brokers has already been one feature of a programme launched by the UK NHS Information Authority (the Electronic Record Development & Implementation Programme (ERDIP) to develop the mechanisms that would allow patients access to their Electronic Health Records (EHR). The Oxford Patient *Access to their online Electronic Health Record (EHR) Project* was one of 18 projects inaugurated in 2000. In the Oxford Patient Access project the IT knowledge brokers (referred to within the project as Information Support Worker) were either seconded from the reception/administrative team or were recruited and trained specifically to work with the patients in this way. The main role of the IT knowledge broker was to introduce patients to their online EHR and help them to develop the skills to access their record securely online without assistance. They also demonstrated links that enabled patients to access additional evidence based health information (Pyper C *et al,* 2001).

Expert knowledge brokers

Disparities in age, educational level, IT skill level, and patient need means that the user requirement for the way knowledge is presented is variable. Expert knowledge brokers are health or social care professionals who utilise their existing skills and develop new information appraisal and communication skills that enable them to make information available in a form palatable to different types of service user. Expert knowledge brokers develop the skills to define a series of user profiles. They work closely with different user groups and identify evidence-based information in a format and at a level that is useful and accessible to that specific user group. In some cases this may involve guidance to appropriate national and local websites, in others a series of information sheets will be more appropriate. The format may be as a leaflet, a website, a CD/DVD, an audio cassette or video, some information will be produced in different languages, larger print or Braille.

A practice nurse with specialist knowledge about diabetes, for example, may work with local diabetic patients, diabetic services and diabetic support groups to clarify the concerns and knowledge requirements of diabetics in different age groups or with different needs – such as learning or language difficulties. Together they will gradually build up and share a database about the different types of diabetic information available and ways of accessing local diabetic NHS networks. In addition they will have access to national recommendations for the management of diabetes including the diabetic Nationals Service Frameworks (NSFs) and information from NICE. A practice nurse working at this level as an expert knowledge broker is likely to have a part-time appointment at a PCT level or across a series of PCTs or at strategic health authority level and share the diabetic database as a website accessible to all the NHS professionals involved in diabetic care. Experience has repeatedly shown that a health database / website such as this needs to be regularly reviewed and updated in order to remain useful to the population it serves. The expert knowledge broker's ongoing role is therefore to be responsible for ensuring the database is monitored, reviewed and amended on a regular basis.

There are further examples of ways in which an expert knowledge broker role may be developed. In 1997 a primary health care team in Oxford identified that they were not adequately managing frequently attending patients whose stress and depression was linked to social or financial problems such as housing, isolation or inability to access benefits. In this case the primary health care team employed a social worker to work within a primary health care team and build an information resource about social services and benefits that complemented the health information. Working with the Community Health Council the primary health care team used fund-holding savings to employ the expert knowledge broker.[4] The knowledge broker saw patients and helped them to access a wide range of information on social, legal, and financial and relationship problems. The project ran for two years and was tremendously popular with the patients. Unfortunately, when fund-holding was abolished, the funding ceased. The evaluation identified the most frequent reasons for patients accessing the service were to receive information or advice about: welfare rights; benefits; social contact and community care. The most frequent users of the service were women living alone over the age of 74 (Pyper *et al*, 2001b). Similar projects have involved Citizens' Advice Bureaux based within General Practice (Galvin *et al,* 1996; Veitch, 1995).

The informal approach adopted by these knowledge brokers involves the development of new skills for networking and learning that can be transferred back to the training needs of the relevant professional groups.

Community knowledge brokers

Community knowledge brokers are people who broker the information exchange between different groups of patients or between patients and professionals whilst being located within the communities that the health services may be trying to reach. They bring with them diverse backgrounds and a skill mix that is far wider than that offered by traditional NHS social services. Their role may involve facilitating interactions among the individuals and groups within a community whose priorities may differ or who may not be equally vocal in articulating their health or social care needs. The skills of the community knowledge broker lie in enabling those individuals or groups who are more isolated and less vocal or confident to articulate their needs and concerns and to work with them to seek solutions that are relevant to them.

The community knowledge brokers will often implicitly acknowledge that they do not have all the answers and facilitate the group to problem solve their own concerns and seek solutions. This process involves recognising that, within large groups, there is a wealth of local knowledge that is often under resourced or valued and alongside this there is minsinformation that requires discussion and clarification. Knowledge brokers enable those they work with to develop the skills to access the knowledge they are seeking, as well as enable them to develop innovative ways to address health or social problems or access services.

Community knowledge workers need training in facilitation skills and the way they work with communities. It takes time to build trust within a community and get a participatory process working. All too often the communities are briefly consulted and the term community participation is used but the participatory element is sheer tokenism. A study exploring the experience of residents involved in urban regeneration projects found that in some cases communities' local interests conflicted with each other (Anastacio *et al,* 2000). Residents felt there was a gap between the rhetoric that demands community participation in area regeneration programmes and the realities of work on the ground. They commented that the mechanisms for community involvement had been inadequate with too little time for effective consultation. They felt there had been insufficient support and training.

Rifkin's review of the community participation in the context of social development and poverty quotes Oakley (1989), identifying three types of participation, recognising the shift in power and decision making from the service providers to the community.

- Marginal participation in which participation is limited in scope and focused on a particular objective: this type has little influence on the community development process
- Substantive participation where beneficiaries have some input determining priorities and contributing to activities and receive benefits but have no role in decision-making: the scope of participation is externally controlled
- Structural participation in which the people play an active and direct role in project development

Muller (1983) makes a distinction between

- Direct participation: implementation of projects through the mobilisation of community resources.
- Social participation: the situation where the community decides and therefore takes control over the factors, which control health

It is the structural participation that the community knowledge brokers are initially trying to facilitate. The process will be to use direct participation with resource implications for the NHS. Over time the more sustainable initiatives will evolve to the social participation model where the community takes more responsibility for communications and the way health and social services are delivered.

One example of the way that this has worked in practice is provided by a multi-centred community participation programme carried out in seven developing countries by International Planned Parenthood Federation with funding from the Department for International Development (DfID). The community participation programme involved family-planning health care providers training to work across the communities and identify their health and other community concerns. The programme was evaluated after three years and again after six years. In the successful sites the local health, social and community services had become more responsive to the needs of their communities. In addition the projects were most sustainable in those situations where the facilitators were members of the community and the community had maintained the process. Often in these cases the community had developed innovative ways to generate long term funding to enable the facilitators to continue their work (Pyper, 1997). A training of experienced trainers initiative allowed

Policy recommendations

> The real voyage of discovery consists not in seeking new lands but in seeing with new eyes
>
> Marcel Proust (1871-1922)

Significant improvements in the health system will not occur without a review of existing practices with the aim of reducing inappropriate demand for health and social care and ensuring that NHS services build closer partnerships with patients and communities. Knowledge brokers could play a key role in securing both of these improvements.

The first step towards development of knowledge broker roles has already taken through the Government's aim of building an integrated IT system. This includes moves to provide access to additional information about health care and evidence-based management via services such as NHS Direct online and the National electronic library. CAREDirect, a further service delivered via NHS Direct, will provide an integrated gateway for older people to get information about, and access to, social care, health, housing and social security benefits.

Where electronic communication systems are being implemented, a role for knowledge brokers is already emerging. The NHS is developing a framework for implementing electronic booking systems using of a variety of interfaces including e-mail, digital TV, call centres and automated reminder booking/broker services. Where the service is developed an IT information broker will be employed to provide the information that patients need to decide when and where they will have their appointment and to enable bookings to be made.

The next step is for the Government to encourage health care organisations use expert knowledge brokers to provide more tailored and appropriate information to their populations; promoting healthy life-style practices, practising self-care for minor conditions and shared management for chronhic conditions thus reducing dependency on health services. The most appropriate organisations for managing and orchestrating this process will be Primary Care Trusts and Strategic Health Authorities who will require pooled resources to support these activities.

However, much of the initiative and identification of need for knowledge brokers, as the examples demonstrated, will come from provider and client organisations. Initiatives to develop a peer knowledge broker or a community knowledge broker, for example, may emerge organically from a particular client group or be initiated by a charity or voluntary organisation. The creation of an Expert knowledge broker may come from a PCT or NHS Trust that is seeking to refine the way that information is provided or to improve the way that they communicate with different patient groups. The first stage will be for NHS bodies or service provider to observe the current way a service is being managed, question assumptions and review the existing procedures.

The next stage, if scope for a broker of knowledge or information is identified, is to question what and whom a new form of service delivery would involve. It is important that all stakeholders, including patients, are involved in the process of consultation from the outset. The process of bringing about change within the organisation is important: it creates a culture that is more reflective and open to the change involved in introducing new knowledge brokers.

Having identified a new way to deliver a service that will involve the knowledge brokers working more closely with patients, the trainee knowledge brokers must be recruited. In most NHS existing workforces there are many individuals with these skills who, at present, are under-utilised and carrying out more didactic roles when they interact with patients. The challenge is to develop effective selection processes that identify these individuals. The skills required by the knowledge brokers are not as specialist as the training required by many health professionals. Knowledge brokers need good communication organisational and IT skills, they need to know how to put people at ease, how to listen and know how to ask open questions and feel comfortable to discuss sensitive subjects.

Once selected, these individuals need an additional training that enables them to develop their knowledge management, facilitation and communication skills. The key skills are understanding how to resource the different knowledge bases available; enable people to articulate and discuss their concerns; respect the varied cultural and health beliefs of the people they are working with and supporting them to make their own decisions. In addition they will need to show patients how to use new technologies to access information systems and secure online services, this will include demonstrating how registration, authentication and consent procedures are implemented.

It is important to identify cost-effective and sustainable training and supervision strategies. The training needs are best met and training existing trainers to acquire these new skills and using a cascade system. Many trainers will already have many of the skills required and will only need about five days additional training. This can be carried out as part of their ongoing professional development. The trainers then need to co-train with more experienced trainers in order to build the confidence to set up their own training programmes.

The training of expert knowledge brokers and IT knowledge brokers can be undertaken by existing professional educators who have gained the additional skills necessary. An existing Nurse Practitioner within a Diabetes Service could, for example, develop additional skills in tailoring information to the needs of his/her patients and use these skills to train additional knowledge brokers, if required. The training of peer knowledge brokers and community knowledge brokers can be done either by trainers of community workers who have gained additional skills to train knowledge brokers and, at a later stage by existing peer knowledge brokers and community knowledge brokers who have acquired training skills.

These training programmes can be delivered as a series of workshops which progress alongside the changes being implemented for service management. Building a learning culture into the working day and having a workshop every one to two weeks to review progress can be a more realistic way to bring about change in the overall work force than sending selected individuals way to study a 50-hour curriculum. The training will also involve the trainee working alongside an experienced knowledge broker. Ongoing peer support can be given using online support / networking and group supervision. The courses need to be accredited and the training offer the knowledge brokers a recognisable qualification within the NHS and social services.

In the early stages of implementing such programmes it is essential that there are some elements of evaluation are used to monitor the progress of both the service changes and the training. Ideally a health economist's evaluations should be an integral part of the evaluation procedure. There are many models that have been developed, especially in developing world countries, where training resources are scarce and cascade-training systems have been used successfully.

Recommendations

- A series of pilot sites for the different types of knowledge broker should be initiated and evaluated. This would be part of the remit of the Modernisation Agency who would facilitate the process and disseminate the findings.
- Developing cost-effective training of trainers programmes that address the selection methods and training and supervision needs of the different knowledge brokers.
- Government action should ensure that the information systems and structures are in place and that as well as ensuring all members of the healthcare workforce are connected to ensure they have been given sufficient in-service training and on going support to use the systems.
- Encouraging PCTs and Primary Care Practices to explore the way in which they are providing health information via their existing services, and to consider developing new approaches that enable consistent access to quality information.

References

Anastacio J (2000) *Reflecting realities: participants' perspectives on integrated communities and sustainable development* Policy Press

Bessell TL, McDonald S, Silagy CA, Anderson JN, Hiller JE and Sansom LN (2002) 'Do Internet interventions for consumers cause more harm than good? A systematic review.' *Health Expectations* 5(1):28-37, 2002 Mar

Department of Health (2000) *Pharmacy in the Future – Implementing the NHS Plan* London: TSO

Galvin K *et al* (1996) *Citizens Advice Bureaux in General Practice: A Pilot Project Evaluation* Institute of Health and Community Studies: Bournemouth University

Muller F (1983) 'Contrasts in community participation: case studies from Peru' in Morley D, Rohde J and Williams G (eds) *Practising Health for All* Oxford: Oxford University Press

Oakley P (1989) *Community Involvement in Health Development* Geneva: WHO

Risk A and Dzenowagis J (2001) 'Review of Internet health information quality initiatives' *Journal of Medical Internet Research* 3(4):E28, 2001 Oct-Dec

Parent F, Coppieters Y, and Parent M (2001) 'Information technologies, health, and ' globalization' : anyone excluded?' *Journal of Medical Internet Research.* 3(1):E11, 2001 Jan-Mar

Pyper C (ed) (1997) *Sexual and Reproductive Health- A New Approach for Communities: Community participation is central to the process of change. -A book for primary health care providers and community groups.* International Planned Parenthood Federation Publication

Pyper C, Amery J, Watson M, Crook C and Thomas B (2001a) *The Patient Access to On-Line Medical Records: Background Report Bury Knowle Health Centre 1996-2001* NHS Information Authority: ERDIP

Pyper C, Amery J, Watson M, Thomas B and Crook C (2001b) *Patient Access to On-line Medical Records, Background Report* NHS Information Authority 2001 (2001-1a-609) http://www.nhsia.nhs.uk/erdip/archive/documents/bury/burycc.doc

Pyper C (1997 & 2000) IPPF Community Participation Approach, Follow-up Evaluation Report. IPPF report 1997 and 2000

Veitch D (1995) *Prescribing Citizens Advice: an evaluation of the work of the Citizens Advice Bureau with Health and Social Service in Birmingham* Birmingham District CABx Ltd.

Acknowledgments: The author would like to thank Dr Muir Gray, Dr Pramilla Senanayake, Dr Alison Hill, Dr Justin Amery, Clair Crook, Dir Marion Watson, Graham Soady, Dr Mary Nichols and Kate Saffin for their support.

Endnotes

1 Globally there are many terms used to describe the knowledge brokers required for 21st century health services workforces who will interact directly with the existing work force, patients and their wider community. These include, 'support workers,' 'health facilitators,' 'change agents' and 'information co-coordinators.'

2 The Oxford, Great Yarmouth and Salford teenagers and young parents participatory website project (funded by BT Higher education award, the DOH Teenage Pregnancy Unit and the Girls Friendly Society) website address is www.Teen4.info

3 This practitioner was known in the practice as the 'Information Support Worker'.